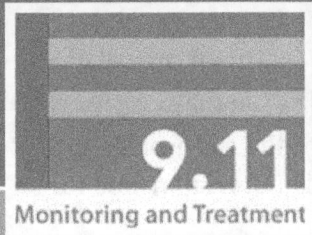

First Periodic Review of Scientific and Medical Evidence Related to Cancer for the World Trade Center Health Program

DEPARTMENT OF HEALTH AND HUMAN SERVICES
Centers for Disease Control and Prevention
National Institute for Occupational Safety and Health

  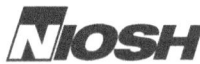

This document is in the public domain and may be freely copied or reprinted.

Disclaimer

Mention of any company or product does not constitute endorsement by the National Institute for Occupational Safety and Health (NIOSH). In addition, citations to Web sites external to NIOSH do not constitute NIOSH endorsement of the sponsoring organizations or their programs or products. Furthermore, NIOSH is not responsible for the content of these Web sites.

Ordering Information

To receive documents or other information about occupational safety and health topics, contact NIOSH at

Telephone: 1–800–CDC–INFO
TTY: 888–533–8573
E-mail: cdcinfo@cdc.gov

or visit the NIOSH Web site at www.cdc.gov/niosh.

For a monthly update on news at NIOSH, subscribe to *NIOSH eNews* at www.cdc.gov/niosh/eNews.

DHHS (NIOSH) Publication Number 2011–197

July 2011

Safer • Healthier • People™

Preface to First Periodic Review of Scientific and Medical Evidence Related to Cancer for the World Trade Center Health Program

The James Zadroga 9/11 Health and Compensation Act of 2010, Public Law 111-347, Title XXXIII of the Public Health Service Act, 124 Stat. 3623 (codified at 42 U.S.C. sec. 300mm—300mm-61), requires the Administrator of the World Trade Center (WTC) Health Program to

> *"periodically conduct a review of all available scientific and medical evidence, including findings and recommendations of Clinical Centers of Excellence, published in peer-reviewed journals to determine if, based on such evidence, cancer or a certain type of cancer should be added to the applicable list of WTC-related health conditions."* 42 U.S.C. sec. 300mm-22(a)(5)(A).

I am pleased to present the first periodic review of cancer for the WTC Health Program.

The review is based on three information sources. First, a systematic search was conducted for peer-reviewed findings on exposure and cancer resulting from the September 11, 2001, terrorist attacks that have been published in the scientific and medical literature between September 11, 2001, and July 1, 2011. Second, findings and recommendations related to cancer were solicited from the WTC Clinical Centers of Excellence and Data Centers, the WTC Health Registry at the New York City Department of Health and Mental Hygiene, and the New York State Department of Health. Third, information from the public about cancer was solicited through a *Request for Information* published in the Federal Register on March 8, 2011, and March 29, 2011.

Overall, this inaugural review of cancer presents findings from the peer-reviewed scientific and medical literature about exposures and cancer resulting from the September 11, 2001, terrorist attacks. In addition, the review provides the status of planned and ongoing research efforts to address questions about cancer related to the exposures resulting from the terrorist attacks.

Specifically, Chapter I describes how the bibliographic search of scientific and medical findings was conducted. Chapter II summarizes the information contained in scientific and medical publications about September 11, 2001, exposures. Chapter III cites the very few peer-reviewed study reports that contain any quantitative data about cancer as a health outcome resulting from September 11, 2001, exposures. In Chapter IV, a primer on cancer epidemiology is presented. In Chapter V, input from the public and from the WTC Clinical Centers of Excellence, the WTC Health Registry, and the New

York State Department of Health about cancer is presented. Chapter VI discusses the challenge of determining whether an observed association between one or more of the September 11, 2001, exposure variables and the health outcome of cancer is causal. Finally, the review includes updates from researchers about current studies of cancer.

It is expected that the second periodic review of cancer will be conducted in early to mid-2012 to capture any emerging findings about exposures and cancer in responders and survivors affected by the September 11, 2001, terrorist attacks.

                                        John Howard, MD
                                Administrator, World Trade Center
                                        Health Program

Acknowledgments

The first periodic review of cancer for the World Trade Center Health Program was researched and developed by the WTC Health Program Cancer Working Group:

Kathleen D. Connick, MSLS, MA
Division of Library Sciences and Services
Office of Surveillance, Epidemiology, and Laboratory Services
Centers for Disease Control and Prevention

Paul Enright, MD
Consultant, NIOSH Division of Respiratory Disease Studies
Professor, School of Medicine
University of Arizona

Paul J. Middendorf, PhD, CIH
National Institute for Occupational Safety and Health
Centers for Disease Control and Prevention

John Piacentino, MD, MPH
National Institute for Occupational Safety and Health
Centers for Disease Control and Prevention

Dori B. Reissman, MD, MPH
National Institute for Occupational Safety and Health
Centers for Disease Control and Prevention

Tamela Sawyer, MS
National Institute for Occupational Safety and Health
Centers for Disease Control and Prevention

Kerry Souza, ScD, MPH
National Institute for Occupational Safety and Health
Centers for Disease Control and Prevention

Appreciation is expressed to the following individuals for their review of the first periodic review of cancer for the WTC Health Program:

Sherry Baron	Kristin Cummings	Gayle DeBord
John Decker	Frank Hearl	Max Kiefer
Ken Martinez	Richard Niemeier	Paul Schulte
Teresa Schnorr	Mary Schubauer-Berigan	Christine Sofge
Douglas Trout	Kenneth Wallingford	David Weissman
Elizabeth Whelan		

Contents

Preface to First Periodic Review of Scientific and Medical Evidence
Related to Cancer for the World Trade Center Health Program.... iii

Acknowledgments v

Abbreviations x

Units of Measurement xii

I. Bibliographic Searches 1
   A. Search Strategies 1
   B. Exposure Results 5
   C. Cancer Results 5
   D. Future Periodic Reviews 5
   E. Other Searches 5

II. Review of Exposures 7
   A. Introduction 7
   B. Designations for Agents Identified at the WTC 8
   C. Environmental Monitoring 9
      1. Chrysotile Asbestos 10
      2. Metals 11
      3. Polychlorinated Polycyclic Compounds 11
      4. Polycyclic Aromatic Hydrocarbons 12
      5. Volatile Organic Compounds 12
      6. Crystalline Silica 13
      7. Fibrous Glass 13
      8. Particulate Matter (Dust) 14
      9. Tritiated Water 14
   D. Biomonitoring 15
      1. Particles Deposited in the Respiratory Tract 15
      2. Metals 15
      3. Polychlorinated Polycyclic Compounds 16
      4. Polycyclic Aromatic Hydrocarbons 16
      5. Volatile Organic Compounds 17
   E. Use of Personal Protective Equipment—Respirators 17
   F. Limitations of Chemical Exposure Assessment 17

G. Other Exposures	18
H. Toxicological Studies	19
III. Review of Cancer	21
A. Cancer Publications	21
B. Peer-Reviewed Cancer Publications	21
1. Risk Models	21
2. Cancer Reviews	21
3. Case Series of Multiple Myeloma	21
C. Non-Peer-Reviewed Cancer Publications	21
1. Letter to the Editor and Author's Response About Multiple Myeloma	21
2. Other	22
IV. Cancer Epidemiology	25
A. Basic Concepts	25
B. Observed Associations and Causal Associations	25
1. Strength	25
2. Consistency	26
3. Specificity	26
4. Temporality	26
5. Biological Gradient	26
6. Plausibility	26
7. Coherence	26
8. Experiment	27
9. Analogy	27
C. Challenges in Establishing Causal Association	27
D. Adding Cancer in the WTC Health Program	28
1. Procedures	28
2. Weighing the Evidence	29
V. Additional Input	31
A. Public Input Opportunities	31
1. Stakeholder Meeting	31
2. Request for Information	31
B. Request for Information Input	32
1. Organizations	32
2. Individuals	33

    C. Input from WTC Clinical Centers of Excellence and the
        WTC Health Registry... 33
        1. Fire Department of the City of New York 34
        2. Mount Sinai School of Medicine................................ 35
        3. World Trade Center Health Registry 36
    D. New York State Department of Health................................ 38

VI. DISCUSSION OF FINDINGS 39
    A. Exposure Publications 39
    B. Cancer Publications... 39
    C. Determination 40

APPENDIX A. REFERENCES 41

APPENDIX B. EXPOSURE PUBLICATIONS............................... 49
    A. Peer-Reviewed 49
    B. Editorials, Abstracts, News Articles (Not Peer-Reviewed) 63

APPENDIX C. CANCER-RELATED PUBLICATIONS AND ARTICLES 75
    A. Peer-Reviewed Publications.................................. 75
    B. Editorial Letters 75
    C. Abstracts, Articles Mentioning Cancer, and Student Thesis 75

APPENDIX D. CANCER CLASSIFICATION SYSTEMS....................... 77
    A. IARC Monographs on the Evaluation of Carcinogenic Risks
        to Humans 77
        Group 1. Carcinogenic to Humans................................. 78
        Group 2A. Probably Carcinogenic to Humans 79
        Group 2B. Possibly Carcinogenic in Humans 79
        Group 3. Not Classifiable as to Its Carcinogenicity to Humans 79
        Group 4. Probably Not Carcinogenic to Humans....................... 79
    B. U.S. National Toxicology Program Report on Carcinogens 80

APPENDIX E. IARC AND NTP DESIGNATIONS FOR
IDENTIFIED CHEMICAL AGENTS 83

Abbreviations

ACS	American Cancer Society
AED	Aerodynamic equivalent diameter
ATSDR	Agency for Toxic Substances and Disease Registry
COPC	Contaminants of potential concern
EPA	Environmental Protection Agency
FDNY	Fire Department of the City of New York
IARC	International Agency for Research on Cancer
IL	Interleukin
MM	Multiple myeloma
MRL	Minimum risk level
NAAQ	National Ambient Air Quality
NIEHS	National Institute of Environmental Health Sciences
NIOSH	National Institute for Occupational Safety and Health
NTP	National Toxicology Program
NYC	New York City
NYCDOHMH	New York City Department of Health and Mental Hygiene
NYSDEC	New York State Department of Environmental Compliance
NYSDOH	New York State Department of Health
OSHA	Occupational Safety and Health Administration
PAH	Polycyclic aromatic hydrocarbon
PCB	Polychlorinated biphenyl
PCM	Phase contrast microscopy
PCDD	Polychlorinated dibenzodioxin
PCDF	Polychlorinated dibenzofuran
PCDD/F	Polychlorinated dibenzodioxins and polychlorinated dibenzofurans
PCM	Phase contrast microscopy
PEL	Permissible exposure limit
PM2.5	Particulate matter with aerodynamic diameter of 2.5 µm or less
PM10	Particulate matter with aerodynamic diameter of 10 µm or less
PM10-53	Particulate matter with aerodynamic diameter between 10 and 53 µm
REL	Recommended exposure limit

RoC	National Toxicology Program 12th Report on Carcinogens
SVF	Synthetic vitreous fiber
TEM	Transmission electron microscopy
TEQ	Toxic equivalents
TNF-α	Tumor necrosis factor-alpha
VOC	Volatile organic compound
WHO	World Health Organization
WTC	World Trade Center
WTC MMTP	World Trade Center Medical Monitoring and Treatment Program

Units of Measurement

f/cm³	fibers per cubic centimeter of air
mg/m³	milligrams per cubic meter of air
ηCi/L	nanoCuries per liter of medium
ηg/m³	nanograms per cubic meter of air
ρg/m³	picograms per cubic meter of air
ppb	parts per billion parts of medium
ppm	parts per million parts of medium
μg/m³	micrograms per cubic meter of air
μm	micrometer

I. Bibliographic Searches

Pursuant to Section 3312(a)(5)(A) of the James Zadroga 9/11 Health and Compensation Act of 2010, a comprehensive and systematic review of the published scientific and medical literature was undertaken to compile a bibliography of peer-reviewed journal publications[1] on exposures resulting from the September 11, 2001, terrorist attacks in New York City and cancer studies in relation to those attacks.

A. Search Strategies

To compile the bibliographies on exposure and cancer, ten bibliographic databases covering biomedical, toxicological, and occupational health information were searched. Although the contents of the databases overlap, each database serves a unique function, has a distinct subject emphasis, and indexes literature not available elsewhere. The databases were chosen on the basis of their content focus and whether they were available on the Internet (PubMed and Toxline), or available through a site license from the Centers for Disease Control and Prevention's Public Health Library & Information Center. The bibliographic databases searched were:

- CISILO (OSH References Collection)
- Cochrane Library
- Embase (OVID)
- Health and Safety Science Abstracts (CSA)
- HSELine (OSH References Collection)
- NIOSHTIC-2 (OSH References Collection)
- OSHLine (OSH References Collection)
- PubMed
- Toxline
- Web of Science

PubMed, Embase, and Health and Safety Science Abstracts can be searched using free-text words in the titles and abstracts and also by using standardized indexing terms (i.e., controlled vocabulary or thesauri) assigned to each record. Initially key articles were identified and reviewed for common text words and search terms that indexers had applied to the articles. These terms were then used to perform the searches and are identified below (see Table 1). The search was not restricted by format; therefore, the returned

---

[1] To determine the peer review status of a journal, the title was searched in Ulrichsweb Global Serials Directory. The Directory contains a basic description of each journal title (publisher, content type, etc.) If a title is peer reviewed, the basic description lists that title as "Refereed." The following are not considered to have peer review status: Commentary; Editorial; Government Report; Letter to the Editor; Meeting Abstract; News Item and Trade Publication.

Table 1. Bibliographic search strategy and results for exposure and cancer

Bibliographic database	Search strategy for cancer	Search strategy for exposure
CISILO (OSH References Collection)	"World Trade Center" OR WTC	"World Trade Center" OR WTC
Cochrane Library	"World Trade Center" OR WTC	"World Trade Center" OR WTC
Embase (Ovid)	#1 World Trade Center [text word] OR WTC [text word] #2 Cancer [text word] OR Neoplasm [subject heading] #1 and #2	(Biological marker OR Air Pollutant OR Air Pollution OR Environmental Monitoring OR Carcinogen OR Occupational Exposure OR Environmental Exposure OR Dust Exposure OR Toxic Inhalation).sh. AND ("World Trade Center" OR "September 11").af. Human, English, not Pub Med
Health and Safety Science Abstracts (CSA)	((World Trade Center) OR WTC) AND DE=(Cancer OR Carcinoma OR (Carcinogenic Agents))	((World Trade Center) OR WTC) AND DE = ((Occupational Exposure) OR Bioindicators OR (Hazardous Materials))
HSELine (OSH References Collection)	("World Trade Center" OR WTC) AND (Cancer OR Neoplasm* OR Carcinogenic OR Carcinoma)	"World Trade Center" AND Exposure*
NIOSHTIC-2 (OSH References Collection)	("World Trade Center" OR WTC) AND (Cancer OR Neoplasm* OR Carcinogenic OR Carcinoma)	("World Trade Center" OR WTC) AND Exposure*

(Continued)

Table 1 (Continued). Bibliographic search strategy and results for exposure and cancer

Bibliographic database	Search strategy for cancer	Search strategy for exposure
OSHLine (OSH References Collection)	("World Trade Center" OR WTC) AND (Cancer OR Neoplasm* OR Carcinogenic OR Carcinoma)	("World Trade Center" OR WTC) AND Exposure*
PubMed	"World Trade Center"[Text Word] OR "September 11 Terrorist Attacks"[Mesh] OR (("Disasters"[MeSH Major Topic] AND "Terrorism"[MeSH Major Topic]) AND ("World Trade Center"[All Fields] OR WTC[All Fields])) AND ("Neoplasms"[Mesh] OR "Carcinogens"[Mesh] OR "Carcinogens, Environmental"[Mesh] OR Cancer[Text Word])	("September 11 Terrorist Attacks"[Mesh] OR ("Disasters"[MeSH] AND "Terrorism"[MeSH] AND "World Trade"[All Fields]) OR ("Disasters"[MeSH] AND "Terrorism"[MeSH] AND WTC[All Fields])) AND ("Biological Markers"[Mesh] OR "Air Pollutants"[Mesh] OR "Environmental Monitoring"[Mesh] OR "Hazardous Substances"[Mesh] OR "Air Pollution"[Mesh] OR "Explosions"[Mesh] OR "Carcinogens"[Mesh] OR "Maternal Exposure"[Mesh] OR "Environmental Exposure"[Mesh] OR "Inhalation Exposure"[Mesh] OR "Occupational Exposure"[Mesh])
TOXLINE	("World Trade Center" OR WTC) AND (Cancer OR Neoplasm* OR Carcinogen* OR Carcinoma)	"World Trade Center" OR WTC OR "September 11" exclude PubMed records

(Continued)

Table 1 (Continued). Bibliographic search strategy and results for exposure and cancer

Bibliographic database	Search strategy for cancer	Search strategy for exposure
Web of Science	"World Trade Center" AND (Cancer OR Carcinogen* OR Neoplasm* OR Carcinoma)	TS="World Trade Center" OR TS="September 11" AND Language=(English)
		Refined by: Subject Areas= (PUBLIC, ENVIRONMENTAL & OCCUPATIONAL HEALTH OR ENVIRONMENTAL SCIENCES OR ENVIRONMENTAL STUDIES OR TOXICOLOGY OR IMMUNOLOGY OR RESPIRATORY SYSTEM)

literature citations include peer-reviewed articles; non-peer-reviewed articles; meeting abstracts; paper proceedings; and academic theses.

The abstract of every citation retrieved was reviewed to determine its relevance to environmental and occupational exposures resulting from the September 11, 2001, terrorist attacks and cancer outcomes. By using the acronym "WTC" in the search strategies, many irrelevant citations were retrieved, and these were disqualified after review. Two separate searches were conducted: (1) a search for publications on environmental and occupational exposures resulting from the September 11, 2001, terrorist attacks; and (2) a search for publications referring to both cancer and the September 11, 2001, terrorist attacks (e.g., searching with "WTC"). Both searches were completed on June 22, 2011.

B. Exposure Results

A total of 294 articles that addressed environmental and occupational exposures resulting from the September 11, 2001, terrorist attacks were returned from the search and review of the literature. Of these 294 articles, 156 are peer-reviewed and 138 are not peer-reviewed publications (see Chapter II and Appendix B).

C. Cancer Results

A total of 18 publications that mention cancer and the September 11, 2001, terrorist attacks were identified as a result of bibliographic searches conducted for this review. See Chapter 1. Of these 18 publications, five addressed environmental monitoring or biomonitoring conducted in response to the September 11, 2001, terrorist attacks, but these publications did not contain any quantitative data concerning cancer as a health outcome. Of the 13 remaining publications, eight were not peer-reviewed and five were peer-reviewed (see Chapter III and Appendix C).

D. Future Periodic Reviews

Two of the databases searched—PubMed and Web of Science—have an automatic alerting service to update and mail search results from a saved search. This feature is being used to enable weekly updates of this bibliography. The other eight databases are searched manually each week and relevant results are added to the bibliography. This systematic review is designed to support periodic reporting on scientific findings related to the health of the exposed population.

E. Other Searches

This review presents scientific and medical evidence "published in peer-reviewed journals" and "findings and recommendations from Clinical Centers of Excellence" as required by law. Data from other sources, such as pension benefit or workers' compensation systems, medical examiners' offices, or similar entities, are not included in this review.

II. Review of Exposures

The scientific literature addressing exposures of individuals who were in the vicinity of the World Trade Center (WTC) in New York City on September 11, 2001, and in the days and weeks afterwards, are discussed in this chapter.

A. Introduction

The destruction of the WTC in Lower Manhattan produced a plume consisting of a unique and complex mixture of chemical agents (including particulates) and exposed a large population of workers and the general public to this mixture. The exposures associated with the September 11, 2001, terrorist attacks were multiple and included physical and chemical agents—some known or reasonably anticipated to be human carcinogens and others not known to be carcinogens—as well as mental and emotional traumatogens. This chapter reviews exposures of a physical or chemical nature, both to known or reasonably anticipated carcinogens as well as other chemicals not known to be carcinogens, and other exposures.

The fires were started by the ignition of 91,000 liters of jet fuel from the two commercial aircraft that crashed into the towers and spread to an estimated 100,000 tons of organic debris, 490,000 liters of transformer oil, 380,000 liters of heating and diesel oil, and fuel from several thousand automobiles which were stored in subterranean structures of the WTC [Pliel et al. 2004]. The plume contained the combustion products of jet fuel, soot, metals, volatile organic compounds, and hydrochloric acid. It also contained particulate matter from pulverized building materials such as cement and glass, as well as building contents, which produced cement dust, glass fibers, asbestos, crystalline silica, metals, polycyclic aromatic hydrocarbons, polychlorinated biphenyls, polychlorinated furans, organochlorine pesticides and dioxins [Lioy 2002; McGee et al. 2003]. As the plume moved away from the towers, particulate and semi-volatile components were deposited for miles around Lower Manhattan, Brooklyn, and beyond. The components and concentrations of the plume likely changed rapidly over the first few hours after the burning and collapse of the WTC towers and as the plume moved away from the epicenter.

Unfortunately, no air sampling devices were operating close to the WTC site to characterize and quantify the constituents of the dust cloud and smoke plumes, and people's exposures to the specific agents and concentrations in the early portions of the disaster will never be known with certainty. After the WTC towers had collapsed, fires in the building rubble continued to burn until December of 2001.

In the days and weeks following the collapse of the WTC towers, numerous agencies, among them the New York City Department of Health and Mental Hygiene (NYCDOHMH), the New York State Department of Health (NYSDOH), the Agency for Toxic Substances and Disease Registry (ATSDR), the National Institute for Occupational Safety and Health (NIOSH), the US Environmental Protection Agency (EPA), the New York State Department of Environmental Conservation (NYSDEC), the United States Geological Survey (USGS), and the Occupational Safety and Health Administration (OSHA), as well as academic researchers and others, collected ambient air samples and settled dust samples to characterize the actual and potential exposures during the disaster response.

The results of many of the collected samples have been included in databases, such as the WTC Environmental Contaminant Database (http://www.wtcreadings.net/wtc/) maintained by the Mailman School of Public Health of Columbia University, which contains data from tens of thousands of samples of outdoor air, bulk dust, indoor air, and indoor air wipes collected shortly before and after September 11, 2001, in NYC and New Jersey.

Exposures during the disaster response have been assessed by a variety of means. Personal air samples were collected from the breathing zones of workers [Breysse et al. 2005; Geyh et al. 2005; Wallingford and Snyder 2001], and biomonitoring for a variety of agents was also conducted on specific populations [Edelman et al. 2003; Fireman et al. 2004; Horrii et al. 2010; Lederman 2008; Tao et al. 2008].

B. Designations for Agents Identified at the WTC

In 2003, an initial list of agents detected in the area around WTC during the disaster response and recovery periods to which people may have been exposed was prepared by the Contaminants of Potential Concern (COPC) Committee of the World Trade Center Indoor Air Task Force Working Group and is called the World Trade Center Indoor Environment Assessment: Selecting Contaminants of Potential Concern and Setting Health-Based Benchmarks.[2]

The list was developed from the chemicals identified from air samples included in four databases used by the COPC Committee [2003] to select contaminants of potential concern and set health-based benchmarks for indoor environments. The four databases were:

- EPA Region 2's database of environmental sampling results, which contains more than 200,000 records on sampling results for 137 agents[3];

---

[2] http://www.tera.org/peer/WTC/COPC%20-%20Benchmark%20Report%20with%20appendices.pdf. Note that this is a large database assembled by the USEPA and centralizes exposure measurements from many different entities.

[3] Only confirmed compounds were included in this list. Measurements for the dioxin and furan compounds were considered one contaminant in this tally, and were screened using a TEQ analysis. TEQ is a dioxin Toxic Equivalent, calculated relative to the most toxic form of dioxin (2,3,7,8-TCDD). Measurements for asbestos were not differentiated by the asbestos minerals, although measurements used different analytical methods and counted different subsets of fiber types and sizes. All measurements for PCBs were considered one contaminant, although the studies reported concentrations under several different groupings of congeners (e.g., total PCBs, Aroclors).

- New York City Department of Health and Mental Hygiene (NYCDOHMH)/ Agency for Toxic Substances and Disease Registry (ATSDR) public health investigation, which includes sampling results from Lower Manhattan of six minerals, 354 air samples from residential buildings, and 32 samples of fibers collected outdoors and analyzed by phase contrast microscopy (PCM);
- New York City Department of Education sampling in schools, which involved samples collected both indoors and outdoors from six schools between September 2001 and June 2002 and includes more than 30,000 records of air sampling results for more than 70 agents; and
- Chattfield and Kominsky's [2001] survey of indoor air quality.

A total of 287 chemicals or chemical groups were identified from the report [COPC 2003], and each of them was checked against the United Nations International Agency on Research on Cancer (IARC) list of agents classified by (1) the IARC monographs, Volumes 1–100, and (2) the United States National Toxicology Program (NTP) 12th Report on Carcinogens. The list and cancer designations are provided in Appendix D.

C. Environmental Monitoring

Environmental monitoring was conducted by collecting samples from the ambient air [Lorber et al. 2007; Olson et al. 2004; Pleil et al. 2004; Pleil et al. 2007; Swartz et al. 2003]; surface samples [Butt et al. 2004; Landrigan et al. 2004; Pleil et al. 2007; Rayne 2005; Rayne et al. 2005]; bulk samples [Lioy et al. 2002; McGee et al. 2003; Offenberg 2004; Pleil et al. 2007; Yiin et al. 2004]; and run-off [Litten et al. 2003] as well as by high-altitude imaging [Clark et al. 2001].

During the rescue and recovery operations, workers at the site were exposed to the combustion products from the fires that intermittently burned in the rubble and to the dust reentrained by rescue and recovery activities and environmental processes. In the September to October 2001 period, workers' exposures in and around the site to the following chemicals were assessed: asbestos, carbon monoxide, chlorodifluoromethane, diesel exhaust, hydrogen sulfide, inorganic acids, mercury and other metals, polycyclic aromatic hydrocarbons, particulates, respirable crystalline silica, and volatile organic compounds [Wallingford and Snyder 2001]. Others characterized truck drivers' exposures to asbestos [Breysse et al. 2005], particulate matter, and volatile organic compounds during the clean-up efforts [Geyh et al. 2005].

In the absence of direct measurements of exposures, particularly during the early stages of the disaster and response, a variety of estimates of exposure or surrogates for exposure have been used. These include the development of algorithms based on the arrival time at the WTC site [Webber et al. 2009]; environmental samples and questionnaires [Herdt-Losavio 2008]; location [Landrigan 2004]; distance and duration [Lederman et al. 2004]; and duration, location, and modeling [Wolff et al. 2005].

In reviewing the published studies that discussed the chemicals and chemical groups found in the various sample types, several general categories of chemical agents, which may include carcinogenic and non-carcinogenic agents, emerge, and they can be categorized as follows: asbestos, metals, polychlorinated polycyclic compounds, polycyclic aromatic hydrocarbons, volatile organic compounds, crystalline silica, and glass fibers. As noted in section A, many of the agents discussed below are not classified as carcinogens and are included in the discussion to present a more complete profile of physical and chemical agent exposures arising from the September 11, 2001, terrorist attacks.

1. Chrysotile Asbestos

Chrysotile asbestos was used extensively to insulate the WTC North Tower, up to the 40th floor [Nicholson 1971]. Many of the collected worker breathing zone, ambient air, and settled dust samples were analyzed for asbestos using either transmission electron microscopy (TEM), which was used to count structures >0.5 µm in length and determine total surface area of these particles, or phase contrast microscopy (PCM), which was used to count particles >5 µm in length and having an aspect ratio ≥3. Fibers <0.25 µm in diameter will generally not be detected by PCM (e.g., NIOSH Method 7400 [NIOSH 1994a]). PCM does not differentiate between asbestos and other fibers since all particles meeting the counting criteria are counted. If confirmation is required, PCM must be used in conjunction with electron microscopy (e.g., NIOSH Method 7402 [NIOSH 1994a]) to differentiate between asbestos and non-asbestos fibers.

The first ambient air samples for asbestos were collected on September 14, 2001. Over the next few months more than 9400 samples were analyzed for asbestos by TEM, and 22 exceeded the Asbestos Hazard Emergency Response Act standard of 70 structures >0.5 µm long per mm^2 [Lorber et al. 2007]. Over 19,000 air samples were collected for asbestos and analyzed using PCM, and 4 exceeded the OSHA permissible exposure limit (PEL)[4] of 0.1 f/cm^3 [Lorber et al. 2007]. However, none of these samples represented breathing zone concentrations in the dust cloud when the WTC towers collapsed.

Of 804 breathing zone and general area air samples collected for asbestos by NYC-DOHMH contractors or NIOSH and analyzed using PCM, countable fibers (aspect ratio ≥3 and length >5 µm) were identified in 45% of the samples. Eighteen of the 25 samples that had >0.10 f/cm^3 were analyzed by TEM to differentiate between asbestos and non-asbestos fibers and found to have <0.10 asbestos f/cm^3. Differential analysis of the fibers on the filters using polarized light microscopy identified the majority of non-asbestos fibers as fibrous glass, gypsum, and cellulose, which were used in the construction of the WTC buildings [Wallingford and Snyder 2001]. Asbestos exposures to truck

---

[4] The OSHA PELs referenced in this report are 8-hour time-weighted average concentrations which are not to be exceeded in a workshift. Many of the PELs were adopted in 1971 based on consensus standards available at that time. PELs issued since then were based on the available information and set at concentrations that were intended to reduce the likelihood of adverse health outcomes as well as be technically and economically feasible.

drivers during two weeks in October and one week in April of 2002 were assessed and found to range from below the limit of detection for TEM to 0.01 structures per cubic centimeter. The results also indicated that the majority of asbestos fibers were chrysotile and <5 μm in length [Breysse et al. 2005].

Settled dust samples and ambient air samples were collected from two locations in Lower Manhattan beginning one week after the September 11, 2001, terrorist attacks and analyzed for asbestos. Trace amounts of chrysotile asbestos fibers were identified by three methods: x-ray diffraction; polarized light microscopy; and analytical TEM. These fibers were found in all six of the settled dust samples at < 0.01% by volume. However, no asbestos fibers were detected in 73 liters of outdoor air sampled at Water Street near the Brooklyn Bridge. No amphibole fibers were identified in the settled dust or air samples [Nolan et al. 2005].

2. Metals

Several metals were identified in the settled indoor and outdoor dust samples, as well as air samples from Lower Manhattan, following September 11, 2001 [COPC 2003]. The most common metals in the PM10-53 WTC dust were calcium, iron, and zinc, but the following metals were also detected in the PM10 fraction of dust: aluminum, antimony, titanium, and magnesium [Landrigan et al. 2004].

Persons caught in the initial dust cloud on September 11th are expected to have experienced short-term exposures to high concentrations of lead, based on analyses of settled dust samples [Lorber et al. 2007]. In late September the concentrations of lead exceeded the EPA's National Ambient Air Quality (NAAQ) standard for lead of 1.5 μg/m^3, but after mid-October air concentrations of lead were similar to typical background concentrations in New York City [Lorber et al. 2007].

Occupational exposures to metals were assessed by collecting air samples in the breathing zones of emergency response workers during response and recovery activities near the disaster site. The samples were analyzed for 27 metals, including the carcinogens arsenic, beryllium, cadmium, chromium, and nickel. Only trace concentrations, well below pertinent NIOSH recommended exposure limits (RELs) and OSHA permissible exposure limits (PELs), were measured in the samples, with one exception. One sample taken on an oxy-acetylene torch cutter had a cadmium concentration of 8.6 μg/m^3, which exceeded the OSHA PEL of 5 μg/m^3 [Wallingford and Snyder 2001]. Additionally, 16 occupational exposure samples were collected for mercury. Concentrations ranged from below the limit of detection for the analytical method to 0.002 mg/m^3, which are substantially less than the NIOSH REL and OSHA PEL [Wallingford and Snyder 2001]. Note that none of these samples were representative of breathing zone concentrations that occurred at the time of the collapse of the WTC towers.

3. Polychlorinated Polycyclic Compounds

Ambient air was monitored for dioxins, which includes 17 polychlorinated dibenzodioxin (PCDD) and polychlorinated dibenzofuran (PCDF) congeners, at and around the

WTC site between September 16 and late November 2001. The results of the samples for these dioxins at the disaster site ranged from 10 to 170 pg/m³, which is substantially greater than the highest ambient levels previously recorded of 1.0 pg/m³ [Lorber et al. 2007]. In contrast, urban dioxin concentrations have been consistently measured at <0.1 pg/m³, while concentrations downwind of incinerators have been measured in the range of 1–5 pg/m³. A month after September 11th, all PCB concentrations near the WTC site were similar to urban background concentrations. By December 2001, dioxin concentrations were similar to typical urban background concentrations.

The amounts of tetra- through octa-chlorinated dibenzo-p-dibenzodioxins and dibenzofurans (PCDD/F) were measured on alcohol wipe samples collected from the exterior windows at seven sites in Lower Manhattan about six weeks after September 11. High amounts of the 2,3,7,8 substituted congeners (e.g., 2,3,7,8-Tetrachlorodibenzo-p-dioxin) were found in the samples [Rayne 2005; Rayne et al. 2005].

4. Polycyclic Aromatic Hydrocarbons

Particle-bound polycyclic aromatic hydrocarbons (PAHs) are among the products of incomplete combustion produced when carbonaceous materials burn. Air samples collected between September 23, 2001, and March 27, 2002, for PM2.5 were assayed for particle-bound PAHs. Predicted concentrations on September 14 for the nine combined PAHs ranged from 1.3 to 5 ng/m³, which are among the highest reported from outdoor sources [Pleil et al. 2004].

Pliel et al. [2004] estimated that PAH air concentrations at the disaster site during the first 200 days were greater than urban background concentrations. PAH concentrations declined, with an estimated 15-day half-life as the WTC fires were extinguished, and approached background ambient levels of 5 ng/m³ in mid-October 2001 [Lorber et al. 2007]. During the first 100 days after September 11 the fires were the predominant source of PAHs. Later, diesel exhaust was the primary source [Pleil et al. 2004].

Twelve air samples were collected on workers in the September to October time frame and analyzed for 16 PAHs. The PAHs were found at trace to small amounts on the samples, and the concentrations did not exceed any pertinent NIOSH RELs or OSHA PELs [Wallingford and Snyder 2001].

Lioy et al. [2002] examined three settled dust samples and analyzed for PAHs in particles <75 µm in diameter. They measured the amount of 40 typical PAHs with higher molecular weights in excess of 200–300 µg/g, and benzo(a)pyrene was measured at 12 to 24 µg/g. Offenberg et al. [2004] found that the relative percentages of several PAH compounds analyzed were similar in indoor and outdoor settled dust samples.

5. Volatile Organic Compounds

Airborne concentrations of 11 volatile organic compounds (VOCs), including the known human carcinogen benzene, were measured by the EPA as 4-minute "grab samples" within smoldering piles near the disaster site, and the results were used to prevent entry of workers when high concentrations were observed [Lorber et al. 2007]. Concentrations exceeding screening benchmarks were found for acetone, benzene, 1,3-butadiene, chloromethane, and ethylbenzene, but not for 1,4-dioxane, ethanol, styrene, tetrahydrofuran, and xylenes. Several 24-hour samples were collected at the perimeter of the disaster site, and the VOC concentrations were typically about 1000 times lower than those measured by the grab samples.

Twenty-four-hour air samples collected for benzene at and within the restricted areas during the first month following September 11, 2001, often exceeded the ATSDR intermediate minimum risk level (MRL) of 4 ppb, and six of the 14 samples were above the detection limit, ranging from 0.7 to 5 ppb, which exceeds the historic average of 0.5 ppb for NYC [Lorber et al. 2007].

Measurements of 14 VOCs were obtained from personal samplers for 12 truck drivers hauling WTC debris in October 2001 and then for five truck drivers in April 2002 [Geyh et al. 2005]. Benzene was detected in all samples, with a maximum of 9 ppb in October and 4 ppb in April. The measured concentrations of other VOCs were considered very low. Seventy-six samples were collected on other workers and analyzed for VOCs. Ethyl benzene, styrene, and toluene were detected at trace amounts in 14 of the 76 samples, but xylene was not detected in any of the air samples [Wallingford and Snyder 2001].

6. Crystalline Silica

Airborne crystalline silica[5] levels were sampled by the EPA at 14 sites between September 27, 2001, and June 20, 2002. Crystalline silica was not present in any of the 159 samples taken at the disaster site, but about 1% of the approximately 1800 samples collected at other sites around the disaster site did contain crystalline silica. The highest concentration measured was 0.03 mg/m^3 [Lorber et al. 2007].

Occupational exposure samples collected for respirable dust were also analyzed for crystalline silica. Of the 18 samples collected by NIOSH between September 18 and October 4, 2001, none contained crystalline silica above the limit of detection for the analytical method [Wallingford and Snyder 2001].

7. Fibrous Glass

Glass fibers, also referred to as slag wool, man-made vitreous fibers (MMVF), or synthetic vitreous fibers (SVFs), constituted 40% of three settled dust samples collected on September 16 and 17 from weather-protected areas [Lioy et al. 2002]. These SVFs may have come from fiberglass insulation, fireproofing, or ceiling tiles in the WTC towers [Rosati 2004].

---

[5] Crystalline silica includes quartz, cristobalite, and tridymite.

The ATSDR collected settled dust samples from inside and outside of apartments in Lower Manhattan in November 2001. Glass fibers were identified by microscopy in 40 of 83 indoor sites and contributed from 2% to 35% of the dust content; and SVFs were detected in 11 of 14 outdoor settled dust samples and contributed from 1% to 72% of the dust sample content [Lorber 2007].

8. Particulate Matter (Dust)

The bulk of the settled dust was determined to originate from cement and gypsum wallboard, both of which consist primarily of non-carcinogenic calcium compounds [Herdt-Losavio 2008]. The range of particle size in the settled dusts was very broad, and 95% of the mass was in particles >53 μm in diameter [Lioy et al. 2002].

Coarse particles, defined as particles having an aerodynamic equivalent diameter (AED) in the range of 10–53 μm and which are preferentially deposited in the nose and upper airways when inhaled, were highly alkaline (pH 9.0–11.0). Particles in the respirable range, defined as those having aerodynamic equivalent diameters ≤10 μm and which are capable of penetrating to the lower airways, and particles in the ultra-fine size range, defined as particles having an aerodynamic equivalent diameter ≤1 μm, were nearly neutral in pH. While only 2% of the overall mass of settled dust was in particles ≤2.5 μm (PM2.5) [Landrigan et al. 2004], the total amount of PM2.5 dust released was estimated at 11,000 tons [Pleil et al. 2004].

To assess occupational exposures, NIOSH collected 18 samples for respirable dust and 36 for total particulates between September 18 and October 4, 2001. None of the samples exceeded the OSHA PELs. Additional monitoring for personal exposures to particulate matter was conducted for 54 truck drivers hauling WTC debris during October 2001 and April 2002. During October the maximum exposure was 1700 μg/m^3 and was found at the disaster site. The median exposure to total dust was 346 μg/m^3 for the truck drivers in October. During April, the highest exposure measured was 195 μg/m^3 and the median exposure was 144 μg/m^3, which were much less than the exposures measured in October [Geyh et al. 2005].

9. Tritiated Water

Traces of tritiated water were detected in a water sample collected from the WTC sewer and in a water sample collected from the basement of Building 6. Likely sources of the tritium include the emergency signs in the planes that crashed into the WTC Towers, weaponry sites containing tritium, and tritium watches carried by the victims. Tritium movement away from the WTC site is expected to have occurred by evaporation and movement with other water sources through the building rubble into the area surrounded by the slurry wall. It was then collected in the PATH train tunnel, where it was pumped out to prevent flooding. The concentrations of tritium were reported to be 0.174 ηCi/L of water in the sewer sample, and a split sample from the basement of Building 6 contained 3.53 ηCi/L and 2.83 ηCi/L. Each of these results is well below the EPA limit in drinking water of 20 ηCi/L [Parekh et al. 2002; Semkow et al. 2002]

D. Biomonitoring

Nine of the available publications on exposure reported the use of biomonitoring to assess WTC-related exposures of specific groups. In reviewing the published studies that discussed biomonitoring of exposures, several general categories of biomarkers emerge, and they can be categorized as follows: particles deposited in the respiratory tract; and a range of chemicals and chemical groups, including metals, polychlorinated polycyclic compounds, polycyclic aromatic hydrocarbons, and volatile organic compounds. An overview of biomonitored exposures to chemical agents in these five categories follows.

1. Particles Deposited in the Respiratory Tract

Several studies have evaluated particles identified in the respiratory tracts of those exposed to the September 11, 2001, terrorist attacks. Ten months after the collapse, induced sputum samples were obtained from 39 Fire Department of the City of New York (FDNY) firefighters who worked in the WTC dust cloud on the morning of September 11, 2001, and compared with samples from firefighters in Tel Aviv to determine whether a unique pattern of inflammation and particulate matter deposition was associated with WTC dust exposure. As determined by scanning electron microscopy, the percentage of particles larger than 2 μm was greater in the induced sputum of FDNY firefighters than in the Tel Aviv firefighters, the particles were more irregularly shaped for the FDNY firefighters, and many more elements (e.g., titanium, zinc, mercury, gold, tin, and nickel) were identified for FDNY firefighters than Tel Aviv firefighters, whose sputum typically contained silica and clays. No asbestos fibers were identified [Fireman et al. 2004].

Rom et al. [2002] reported the results of bronchoalveolar lavage (BAL) concentrations of a firefighter exposed from September 11 to September 24, 2001, to high concentrations of WTC dust. Mineralogical analysis of the cell pellet obtained by BAL counted 305 asbestos (chrysotile and amosite) fibers/106 macrophages, including those with high aspect ratios, and significant quantities of fly ash and degraded fibrous glass. Another study evaluated particles found in lung tissue of exposed individuals. Case reports of seven previously healthy WTC workers who developed interstitial lung disease identified aluminum and magnesium silicates in unusual platy (sheet) structures, chrysotile asbestos, calcium phosphate and calcium sulfate, small shards of glass, and carbon nanotubes of various sizes and lengths in the lung biopsies of some of these workers (probably due to high-temperature combustion) [Wu et al. 2010].

2. Metals

Concentrations of several metals were measured in samples of blood and urine obtained from 318 FDNY firefighters during the first week of October 2001 who responded to the

WTC disaster, and for 47 firefighters who did not respond and were used as a control group [Edelman et al. 2003]. The authors report that for the WTC responder group, the mean urine concentrations of lead, antimony, cadmium, and uranium and the mean blood concentration of cadmium were greater than for the control group, but below clinically significant levels.

A study was conducted to ascertain the concentrations of mercury in the cord blood of infants whose mothers were pregnant and worked or lived within 1 or 2 miles of the WTC during the WTC disaster and response. The mercury concentrations in cord blood were not elevated in comparison with those of infants whose mothers lived and worked farther away [Lederman et al. 2008].

3. Polychlorinated Polycyclic Compounds

Heptachlorodibenzodioxin and heptachlorodibenzofuran congeners are produced by burning plastics containing chlorine. The concentrations of these compounds in blood samples of WTC-exposed FDNY firefighters were significantly elevated above those for a control group of firefighters. One heptachlorodibenzodioxin congener was significantly elevated in the blood samples of Special Operations Command firefighters and the other firefighters who responded, in comparison with levels in the control group [Edelman et al. 2003].

Concentrations of PCDDs, PCDFs, PCBs, and polychlorinated naphthalenes were measured in the blood of New York State employees and National Guard personnel who worked in the vicinity of the WTC during the week after the collapse of the buildings. Individuals' exposures were estimated and categorized as more or less dust exposure, and more or less smoke exposure. The results indicate that workers in the "More Dust Exposure" and "More Smoke Exposure" categories were more exposed to PCDFs, while the workers categorized as "Less Dust Exposure" or "Less Smoke Exposure" were more exposed to PCDDs [Horii et al. 2010].

4. Polycyclic Aromatic Hydrocarbons

PAH metabolites were measured during the first week of October 2001 in samples of blood and urine obtained from 318 WTC-exposed FDNY firefighters and 47 control firefighters who were not exposed at the WTC [Edelman et al. 2003]. Mean blood or urinary concentrations of all eight PAHs measured from the 95 Special Operations Command firefighters who arrived earliest at the disaster site were significantly greater than for the control firefighters.

In a study of NYC women who were pregnant on September 11, 2001, PAH-DNA adduct concentrations were measured in cord blood and maternal blood [Perera et al. 2005a;b]. Of those women who smoked cigarettes during their pregnancy, those living closest to the disaster site had higher concentrations of PAH-DNA adducts when compared to those living farther away.

5. Volatile Organic Compounds

The mean blood concentrations of xylenes were significantly higher in exposed FDNY firefighters when compared to a control group [Edelman et al. 2003]. Concentrations of eight perfluorochemicals were measured in the blood of 458 New York State and National Guard employees assigned to WTC work after September 11th. The average concentrations were about twice those found in the general U.S. population [Tao et al. 2008].

E. Use of Personal Protective Equipment—Respirators

In the early days of the response, respirator use was considered a paramount issue. However, few studies address the use of respirators, and even fewer studies provide detailed information on types of respirators used. In a study of factors associated with skin, eye, respiratory, nose, and throat symptoms, firefighters who responded were asked to identify from a list of four types of respirators the type they used during five time periods. The four types were: full face mask self-contained breathing apparatus; N95 filtering face mask; half-face elastomeric respirator with combination P-100 and organic vapor/acid gas cartridges; and hardware store–type disposable dust/paint masks that may or may not have been NIOSH-certified and were not fit-tested or fit-checked.

An evaluation of the overall use of respiratory protection among these firefighters during the first two weeks at the WTC site showed that 19% of the study firefighters reported not using a respirator, and 50% reported using a respirator but only rarely [Feldman et al. 2004].

Ninety-six ironworkers who started working at the site between September 11 and September 15 were questioned about their use of respirators, and 41 reported they did not wear a respirator during the first week. Additionally, 33 reported wearing a dust respirator during the first week, and 17 reported wearing a respirator with a canister[6] only during the first week [Skloot et al. 2004].

F. Limitations of Chemical Exposure Assessment

A large number of ambient air and settled dust samples were collected within the first months after the September 11, 2001, terrorist attacks, but relatively few personal air samples or biomonitoring samples were collected. Ambient area air sampling, which comprises most of the air sampling associated with the September 11, 2001, terrorist attacks, is not generally considered to be standard practice for determining exposures among workers.

Additionally, the lack of any environmental or personal samples during the very early stages of the September 11, 2001, disaster, when exposures were the most intense, causes

---

[6] The type of respirator and the type of canister were not identified.

a significant gap in the characterization of exposures. Despite these limitations, a number of exposure assessments based on the collected samples were developed and published in the scientific literature. These assessments suggest that some individual responders were potentially exposed to one or more of the chemicals designated by IARC and NTP as known or reasonably anticipated human carcinogens. Furthermore, the exposure assessments generally focused on narrow categories of chemical agents, identified in air samples or settled dust. The toxicologic significance of complex mixtures of various known occupational carcinogens and other chemical agents is poorly understood. Issues of association between exposure and cancer are discussed in Chapter IV.

G. Other Exposures

In general, the role of exposures other than chemical exposures in the development of cancer is less well-defined. Studies conducted following the September 11, 2001, terrorist attacks did address a few non-chemical agent exposures. Most of these studies addressed exposures in relation to mental and emotional health. Some of those studies are summarized in this section.

Numerous studies have investigated stress-related outcomes (e.g., anxiety, depression, and post-traumatic stress disorder, or PTSD) and exposure to the disaster-related events of the September 11, 2001, terrorist attacks. Many of the studies addressed exposure by the simple metric of proximity to the event [Galea et al. 2003]. Other exposure metrics used include: knowing someone who died; knowing someone who was injured; financial impact; involvement in rescue and/or recovery; knowing someone involved in the rescue and/or recovery [Calderoni et al.; Adams et al. 2005]; being on a high floor in the towers; initiating evacuation late; being caught in the dust cloud that resulted from the tower collapses; personally witnessing horror; sustaining an injury [DiGrande et al. 2011]; and in utero exposure [Endara et al. 2009].

Specifically, PTSD as a health outcome from the terrorist attacks has been extensively studied. In a survey study done in 2003–2004, the prevalence of probable PTSD was 12.6% and was associated with older age, female gender, Hispanic ethnicity, low education and income, and divorce [DiGrande 2008]. And evidence for persisting PTSD has been reported [Neria 2010].

Finally, the role of organizational factors in health outcomes after the terrorist attacks was addressed in one study [Osinubi et al. 2008]. Exposures were assessed using location as the exposure surrogate—workers south of Canal Street were categorized as primary victims, and workers north of Canal Street were categorized as victims or non-victims. The association of these exposures with workers' health and productivity was assessed. A defensive organizational culture was found to be an independent predictor of cough and job stress, and job stress was an independent predictor of productivity loss.

H. Toxicological Studies

Numerous studies evaluated the effects on dogs of exposure at the WTC during rescue and recovery. Each of the studies evaluated respiratory effects and observed no lasting effects [Fox et al. 2008; Otto et al. 2010; Otto et al. 2004; Fitzgerald et al. 2008]. However, dogs deployed at the WTC had a combined morbidity, defined as one or more abnormalities of body systems including traumatic injuries, 6.6 times greater than those deployed at the Pentagon [Slensky et al. 2004]. Also, mild but significant increases were identified for blood serum concentrations of globulin and bilirubin, as well as alkaline phosphatase activity, in WTC-exposed dogs, which was suggestive of higher antigen or toxin exposure [Otto 2004].

A few animal model and in vitro studies have been performed using WTC dusts to investigate the underlying mechanisms of the respiratory responses observed in responders and others. The identified studies have addressed inflammatory responses to the WTC dust, but have not addressed cancer as an outcome.

Fallen dust samples were collected within 0.5 miles of the WTC and size-separated to produce a PM2.5 fraction (derived WTC dust). Mice exposed by aspiration to a relatively high dose of these derived samples showed only moderate pulmonary inflammation but marked bronchial hyperresponsiveness. Lower doses by aspiration or nose-only did not produce significant inflammation or hyperresponsiveness. The results indicate that exposure to high levels of WTC dust can promote mechanisms of airflow obstruction in mice. Airborne concentrations of derived WTC dust that would cause similar effects in humans are estimated to be 425 µg/m^3 for eight hours. The authors concluded that a high-level exposure to WTC PM2.5 could cause pulmonary inflammation and airway hyperresponsiveness in humans [Gavett et al. 2003].

The effects of several size fractions derived from WTC indoor or outdoor dust samples on human primary alveolar macrophages, and type II epithelial cells, which play important roles in defending the lung from the effects of inhaled particles, have been studied. In the primary alveolar macrophages, cytokines (i.e., interleukin [IL]-8, IL-6, and tumor necrosis factor-alpha [TNF-α]) were released at two of the lower concentrations, but fell at the highest concentration. Type II epithelial cells did not release TNF-α, and the releases of IL-8 and IL-6 were lower than in the alveolar macrophages. These findings demonstrate that respirable WTC particulate matter stimulates inflammatory mediator release by lung cells, which might contribute to respiratory illness [Payne et al. 2004]. Further study of cytokine production indicates that the mitogen-activated protein kinase signaling pathway is activated in a dose-dependent manner by WTC dusts, and likely played an important role in the production of inflammatory cytokines [Wang et al. 2010].

III. Review of Cancer

A. Cancer Publications

A total of 18 publications that mention cancer in human subjects and the September 11, 2001, terrorist attacks were identified as a result of bibliographic searches conducted for this review. See Chapter 1. Of these 18 publications, five addressed environmental monitoring or biomonitoring conducted in response to the September 11, 2001, terrorist attacks, but these publications did not contain any quantitative data concerning cancer as a health outcome. Of the 13 remaining publications, eight were not peer-reviewed and five were peer-reviewed.

B. Peer-Reviewed Cancer Publications

The five peer-reviewed scientific and medical publications appear in Table 2 and are summarized below:

1. Risk Models

Two articles used models to estimate the risk of cancer among residents of Lower Manhattan. One of the modeling publications noted a "slightly elevated" risk of cancer [Rayne 2005] and the other modeling publication noted a "negligible" risk of cancer associated with potential exposure to asbestos [Nolan et al. 2005].

2. Cancer Reviews

Two articles were reviews of cancer associated with the September 11, 2001, terrorist attacks [Moline et al. 2006; Samet et al. 2007]. Neither author's review of the literature revealed any epidemiologic evidence for a causal association between September 11, 2001, exposures and cancer, but the authors of both reviews did recommend that monitoring of the responder and survivor populations continue and that cancer screening be considered.

3. Case Series of Multiple Myeloma

One article was a small case series on the diagnosis of cancer in individuals affected by the September 11, 2001, terrorist attacks [Moline et al. 2009]. In a case series of multiple myeloma in eight responders to the September 11th attacks in New York City, the authors observed that the number of multiple myeloma cases in men under the age of 45 (n=4 in the case series) was greater than the authors expected.

C. Non-Peer-Reviewed Cancer Publications

1. Letter to the Editor and Author's Response About Multiple Myeloma

One article was a letter to the editor which noted that the four cases reported by Moline et al. were all law enforcement officers who may have had other occupational exposures that contributed to the development of multiple myeloma [Miller 2009].

One article was a response to the letter to the editor in which the authors agreed that the occurrence of the four cases of multiple myeloma in young responders did not prove causation and recommended continued follow-up of the responder population [Moline et al. 2009b].

2. Other

The remaining four non-peer-reviewed articles mention cancer but do not address cancer as an outcome.

Table 2. Publications and articles related to peer-reviewed publications on cancer

Author/year	Study design	Cohort/geography under study	Study results	Cancer finding
Moline et. al. 2009a	Case series	8 Registered WTC responders (law enforcement)	Multiple myeloma elevated above expected in WTC responders under 45 years of age; no epidemiologic analysis conducted	Greater than expected # cases of multiple myeloma
Miller 2009	Letter to the editor	Moline et. al. 2009	Response to Moline 2009 paper, noting potential biases and selection issues	N/A
Moline et. al. 2009	Response to letter to the editor	Moline et. al. 2009	Response to Miller, 2009, re: potential bias and selection issues	N/A
Moline et. al. 2006	Review article	WTC responders	Review of short and medium term health effects and review of WTC exposures; author recommended screening of cohort for cancer	N/A

(Continued)

Table 2 (Continued). Publications and articles related to peer-reviewed publications on cancer

Author/ year	Study design	Cohort/geography under study	Study results	Cancer finding
Samet et. al. 2007	Comment	N/A	Reviews types and quantities of dust/particulates likely present following 9/11/2001, and evidence of exposures. Discussion of uncertainties involved and need to follow cohorts to monitor for long-term cancer risk.	N/A
Rayne 2005	Environmental survey/ Risk assessment	Lower Manhattan	Based on window film sampling 6 weeks following WTC attacks, author estimates that Lower Manhattan residents have a slightly elevated cancer risk due to exposures to certain semi-volatile organic compounds	Increased cancer risk predicted by risk assessment
Nolan et. al. 2005	Risk assessment	WTC environmental sampling	Cancer risk associated with assumed asbestos exposures for residents of Lower Manhattan resulting from the collapse of the WTC is negligible.	Estimated excess risk of 1 case of cancer for Lower Manhattan residents

IV. Cancer Epidemiology

A. Basic Concepts

The branch of science that deals with the study of the causes, distribution, and control of disease in populations is called epidemiology. The point of many epidemiological studies is to examine or "observe" any associations between an exposure variable, or variables, and health outcome. Unlike studies done in a laboratory, or under controlled conditions, most epidemiological studies are not experimental; they are "observational studies." Such studies are conducted in an inherently "noisy" environment in free-living populations [Lucas 2005]. Chance, bias, and confounding are ever present threats in any epidemiological study and complicate drawing a causal inference from observing an association between exposure and disease. An observed association may not be a causal one.

B. Observed Associations and Causal Associations

Drawing causal inferences about exposures resulting from the September 11, 2001, terrorist attacks and the observation of cancer cases in responders and survivors is especially challenging since cancer is not a rare disease. In the United States, the probability that a person will develop cancer during their lifetime is one in two for men and one in three for women [ACS 2010]. This "background" rate of cancer development would be expected in responders and survivors even if the September 11, 2001, terrorist attacks had never occurred. Determining, then, if the September 11, 2001, exposures are contributing to an additional burden of cancer in responders and survivors is a scientific challenge.

One of the most important frameworks that epidemiologists often use to assess the causal nature of an observed association is the "Bradford Hill criteria" [Hill 1965]. Although published 46 years ago, the Bradford Hill criteria have been described as an important "aid to thought" by the noted epidemiologist who determined that the association between tobacco smoking and lung cancer was a causal one [Doll 2002].

Hill did not propose the criteria as a rigorous checklist, but they are often viewed in that way. The criteria have been criticized as failing to deliver on being able to clearly distinguish causal from non-causal associations [Rothman 2002]. None of the nine Bradford Hill criteria are alone sufficient to establish causation, but together they can provide a starting point in evaluating whether an observed association is indeed a causal one. The following sections describe the nine Bradford Hill criteria:

1. Strength

The strength of the association refers to the magnitude of the association between a risk factor and the health effect. Bradford Hill thought that the weak associations were less likely to be causal than strong ones. In contemporary epidemiology, weak associations are often encountered, and much attention needs to be focused on (1) a strong study design and methodology that minimizes bias, (2) evaluation of the role of chance, and (3) measurement of possible confounders of a valid measure of association [Lucas and McMichael 2005].

2. Consistency

Consistency of findings means that you can have more confidence in a causal explanation for an observed association if studies in different populations of similarly exposed individuals show similar health effects. Lack of consistency, though, is not a necessary criterion for a causal interpretation; lack of consistency may provide insights that warrant further investigation [Lucas and McMichael 2005].

3. Specificity

Specificity refers to the idea that any exposure gives rise to only a single outcome [Lemen 2004]. This is generally true for acute communicable diseases—for example, the rubella virus cause only rubella (the disease)—but it is not generally true for non-communicable diseases such as environmental exposures [Lucas and McMichael 2005].

4. Temporality

Temporality means that the exposure precedes the development of the health effect and is viewed as a necessary criterion for determining that an association is causal. There is universal agreement that temporality is truly a causal criterion [Rothman 2002].

5. Biological Gradient

Biological gradient means that the higher the "dose" of exposure, the greater the magnitude or likelihood of the health effect observed. Although useful for a toxicological laboratory experiment, such a quantitative relationship may be a challenge to demonstrate with environmental exposures [Rothman 1998]. Suggestions have been made to develop a new framework for a unified approach to dose-response assessment in environmental risk assessment [NRC 2009].

6. Plausibility

Plausibility means that the exposure–health outcome association makes biologic sense and does not conflict with generally known facts. However, the biological knowledge of the moment may not be sound and may merely reflect prior beliefs—not biologic fact.

7. Coherence

Coherence and biological plausibility share a common judgment that the causal association "fits" with known facts about the biology of the disease.

8. Experiment

Experiment asks the question: If exposure is reduced by preventive actions (e.g., tobacco smoking cessation), does the rate of lung cancer decrease? Public health interventions are designed to reduce or eliminate a hazardous exposure, thereby improving the health outcome associated with that exposure. A positive intervention provides good evidence that the exposure–health outcome association was indeed a causal one.

9. Analogy

Reasoning by analogy is a weak method for identifying associations, but it may have limited use in helping to assess whether an association is a causal one. Exposure to environmental tobacco smoke and the risk of lung cancer can be analogized from the known risk of lung cancer in active smokers [Lucas and McMichael 2005].

C. Challenges in Establishing Causal Association

From a scientific perspective, the task of establishing a causal association between the September 11, 2001, exposures and cancer poses some challenges for a number of reasons.

When the particular health effect is highly prevalent in the population, it takes more effort to distinguish causation arising from just one type of exposure. As stated above, because cancer is not a rare disease in the United States, many cases of cancer are expected to occur in any subset of the American population, regardless of exposures resulting from the terrorist attacks. Observing a disproportionate number of cases of cancer than the number expected would be an important finding in WTC cancer studies.

Many exposures associated with cancer (e.g., smoking, diet, and genetic influences) are not unique to a single event in the individual's life (like the September 11, 2001, terrorist attacks), making it more challenging to draw a causal association between cancer and just one of those exposures. The assessment of multifactor causation is a special challenge to cancer epidemiology.

When the observation period is shorter than the average time that it takes for cancer to develop biologically following exposure (i.e., latent period), an excess of cancer cases would not be expected to be seen.

An important feature of cancer epidemiology is being able to represent exposure quantitatively. The limitations of the WTC exposure assessment literature as discussed in Chapter II make precise quantitative (e.g., breathing zone) exposure assessment a challenge, and qualitative categories may be utilized (e.g., time of arrival, duration of response or recovery work, and proximity to the dust cloud). This is often the case when assessing "real world" environmental exposures.

D. Adding Cancer in the WTC Health Program

1. Procedures

Section 300mm-22(a)(5)(A) of Title XXXIII of the Public Health Service Act, codifying the James Zadrogra 9/11 Health and Compensation Act of 2010, ("Act"), requires the Administrator of the WTC Health Program to conduct periodically a review of all available scientific and medical evidence published in peer-reviewed journals for the purpose of determining if, based on that evidence, cancer or a certain type of cancer should be added to the List of WTC-Related Health Conditions ("List") found in Section 300mm-22(a)(3) and 300mm-32(b).

The Act further specifies that if the Administrator determines that cancer or a certain type of cancer should be added to the List, the Administrator shall propose the addition(s) through rulemaking. Based on all available evidence in the rulemaking record, the Administrator shall make a final determination of whether cancer or a certain type of cancer should be added to the List and promulgate a rule to that effect, or publish an explanation for why cancer or a certain type of cancer should not be added to the List. *See* 42 U.S.C. sec. 300mm-22(a)(5)(B) through (D).

In Section 300mm-22(a)(6), the Act provides that whenever the Administrator determines that a proposed rule should be promulgated to add any type of health condition (including cancer or a certain type of cancer) to the List, the Administrator may either (1) request a recommendation of the WTC Health Program Scientific/Technical Advisory Committee ("STAC") or (2) publish a proposed rule in the Federal Register.

The Act also provides for the receipt of written petitions by an interested party to add a health condition to the List. An interested party is defined in Section 300mm-22(a)(6)(E) and "includes a representative of any organization representing WTC responders, a nationally recognized medical association, a Clinical or Data Center, a State or political subdivision, or any other interested person."

In the case of a petition to add a health condition to the List, the Administrator not later than 60 days after the date of receipt of the petition shall do one of the following: (1) request a recommendation from the WTC Health Program STAC; (2) publish in the Federal Register a proposed rule to add such a health condition to the List; (3) publish in the Federal Register a determination not to propose a rule adding the health condition; or (4) publish in the Federal Register a determination that insufficient evidence exists to take any of these actions. *See* 42 U.S.C. sec. 300mm-22(a)(6)(B).

If the Administrator of the WTC Health Program requests a recommendation from the WTC Health Program STAC, the WTC Health Program STAC is required to submit to the Administrator its recommendation not later than 60 days after the date of the Administrator's request or by a date (not to exceed 180 days after the Administrator's request) specified by the Administrator.

Not later than 60 days after receiving the recommendation from the WTC Health Program STAC, the Administrator shall (1) publish a proposed rule regarding the recommendation; or (2) publish the Administrator's determination in the Federal Register not to publish a proposed rule and the basis for such determination. *See* 42 U.S.C. sec. 300mm-22(a)(6)(C).

2. Weighing the Evidence

In addition to specifying the procedures for adding health conditions, including cancer, to the List, the Act also spells out the basis upon which a determination to add a health condition to the List must be made.

Section 300mm-22(a)(5)(B) provides that the Administrator's determination is "based on the periodic reviews …". Section 300mm-22(a)(5)(A) describes the materials to be included in the periodic reviews and provides the basis for the Administrator's determination on whether to add cancer or a certain type of cancer, as "all available scientific and medical evidence, including findings and recommendations of the Clinical Centers of Excellence, published in peer-reviewed journals…". *All* available scientific and medical evidence is a broad category, but the Act narrows the broad category to include *only* the scientific and medical evidence that is published in peer-reviewed journals.

The Act does not provide specific guidance, though, about how peer-reviewed scientific and medical evidence is to be evaluated or "weighed" by the Administrator in making a determination to add, or not to add, a health condition to the List. "Weight of the evidence" is a common term in the risk assessment literature, but it can have different meanings and applications [Weed 2005]. Some Federal statutes provide more specific guidance on how evidence is to be weighed than the Act does.[7]

---

[7] In the Persian Gulf War Veterans Act (38 U.S.C. §1118), the Secretary of Veterans Affairs is tasked with determining whether a health condition warrants a presumption of service connection by reason of having a positive association with a set of exposures. The determination is one "based on sound medical and scientific evidence that a positive association exists between" specified exposures and an illness in humans or animals. In making the determination, the Secretary must take into account reports submitted by the National Academy of Sciences, all other sound medical and scientific medical information and available analyses. In evaluating any report, information or analysis, the Secretary is required to take into consideration whether the results are statistically significant, are capable of replication, and withstand peer review. An association between exposure and illness shall be considered positive if the credible evidence for the association is equal to or outweighs the credible evidence against the association. See also IOM 2009 and IOM 2010.

V. Additional Input

A. Public Input Opportunities

1. Stakeholder Meeting

On March 3, 2011, NIOSH held a public meeting in New York City to receive comments from the public on implementing the provisions of the James Zadroga 9/11 Health and Compensation Act of 2010. During the meeting, over 40 individuals spoke either in person or by telephone, providing their perspectives on the current program as well as their ideas for how the program should move forward. One of the issues raised during the meeting included the inclusion of cancer into the List of WTC-Related Health Conditions.

See http://www.cdc.gov/niosh/docket/archive/docket226.html for more information about the stakeholder meeting and to access electronic copies of all the submissions to the meeting docket as well as a full transcript of the meeting. A number of submissions to the stakeholder meeting docket addressed cancer.

2. Request for Information

NIOSH announced a Request for Information about cancer in the Federal Register on March 8, 2011 (Vol. 76, No. 45, page 12,740), and amended that Request on March 29, 2011 (Vol. 76, No. 60, page 17,421). NIOSH requested information from the public on the following three questions regarding conditions relating to cancer for consideration under the WTC Health Program:

1. Relevant reports, publications, and case information of scientific and medical findings where exposure to airborne toxins, any other hazard, or any other adverse condition resulting from the September 11, 2001, terrorist attacks is substantially likely to be a significant factor in aggravating, contributing to, or causing cancer or a type of cancer;

2. Clinical findings from the Clinical Centers of Excellence providing monitoring and treatment services to WTC responders and community members directly exposed to the dust cloud, gases, and vapors on September 11, 2001, and those living and working in the affected area; and

3. Input on the scientific criteria to be used by experts to evaluate the weight of the medical and scientific evidence regarding such potential health conditions.

NIOSH received ten submissions from the public, which are published in the NIOSH Docket (see Docket 227 at http://www.cdc.gov/niosh/docket/archive/docket227.html).

NIOSH thanks all those who submitted comments on conditions related to cancer for the WTC Health Program. The submissions can be divided into two general categories: (1) submissions by organizations and (2) submissions by individuals.

B. Request for Information Input

1. Organizations

- Uniformed Firefighters Association (UFA) noted the growing number of firefighters that are being diagnosed with cancers such as non-Hodgkin's lymphoma and multiple myeloma and that these conditions need to be added for coverage in the World Trade Center Health Program. A separate submission reviewed the biological plausibility of chemical synergism as an underlying mechanism promoting the development of cancer in the WTC responders.

  http://www.cdc.gov/niosh/docket/archive/pdfs/NIOSH-227/0227-042811-Royce_sub.pdf

  http://www.cdc.gov/niosh/docket/archive/pdfs/NIOSH-227/0227-032811-Romaka_sub.pdf

- NYS Laborers Health and Safety Trust Fund requested that NIOSH consider three sources of information to inform scientific criteria to weigh the evidence. These are (a) the exposures experienced by WTC responders and survivors and the scientific literature on cancer related to these exposures; (b) general knowledge of cancers related to exposure to chemicals and toxins; and (c) follow-up studies of WTC responders and survivors.

  http://www.cdc.gov/niosh/docket/archive/pdfs/NIOSH-227/0227-033111-Melius_sub.pdf

- International Myeloma Foundation (IMF) provided background information on myeloma, including research linking myeloma with environmental exposures; and requested an aggressive outreach campaign.

  http://www.cdc.gov/niosh/docket/archive/pdfs/NIOSH-227/0227-042911-Durie_sub.pdf

- The Patrolmen's Benevolent Association of the City of New York, Inc. (PBA) requested the addition of multiple myeloma to the list of covered conditions for treatment, given the research evidence [Moline 2009]. The letter also suggests that the WTC Program Administrator evaluate evidence and exercise discretion in adding additional types of cancer such as those that appear more frequently within the responder population.

  http://www.cdc.gov/niosh/docket/archive/pdfs/NIOSH-227/0227-042911-Tramontano_sub.pdf

- NYC Department of Health and Mental Hygiene submitted the 2010 Annual Report from New York City's World Trade Center Medical Working Group, which reviews the WTC health effects literature and recommends specific standard methodological approaches to assist the future comparison of studies regarding WTC exposure and cancer.

http://www.cdc.gov/niosh/docket/archive/pdfs/NIOSH-227/0227-042811-Farley_sub.pdf

2. Individuals

- A member of the public asked NIOSH to change the original Federal Register request for information on WTC cancer to include those who lived, worked, or attended schools in the impacted neighborhoods in the days, weeks, and months following the attack.

  http://www.cdc.gov/niosh/docket/archive/pdfs/NIOSH-227/0227-031011-Polett_sub.pdf

- A member of the public submitted a review of the historical investigations of Agent Orange and the Gulf War Syndrome in evaluating chemical injury and the harm from inappropriate diagnoses. A clinical algorithm was suggested for the evaluation of the chemically injured patient to help differentiate physical from psychosomatic injury after toxic chemical exposure.

  http://www.cdc.gov/niosh/docket/archive/pdfs/NIOSH-227/0227-042911-Moore_sub.pdf

- A member of the public submitted two lengthy reports—Report Docket No. NIOSH 227 JP and JP2—about the causes of the September 11, 2001, events in New York City in relation to the development of human cancers.

  http://www.cdc.gov/niosh/docket/archive/pdfs/NIOSH-227/0227-031411-Prager_sub.pdf

  http://www.cdc.gov/niosh/docket/archive/pdfs/NIOSH-227/0227-031511-Prager_sub.pdf

C. Input from WTC Clinical Centers of Excellence and the WTC Health Registry

The WTC Program Administrator sent a letter on June 3, 2011, to the WTC Data Centers, WTC Clinical Centers of Excellence, and the WTC Health Registry requesting information relevant to this review.

In the June 3, 2011, letter, the Administrator noted that the review would be greatly enriched by (1) any clinically observed findings, including trends, that are unpublished, but which are believed to be important clinical observations pertaining to cancer; (2) any planned data analysis or research efforts pertaining to cancer; and (3) any findings pertaining to cancer that are being prepared for publication, with an estimate of when such paper(s) are expected to be published.

The Administrator received submissions from the Fire Department of the City of New York, the Mount Sinai School of Medicine, and the New York City Department of Health and Mental Hygiene's World Trade Center Health Registry.

1. Fire Department of the City of New York (FDNY)[8]

FDNY researchers, in collaboration with the FDNY WTC Clinical Center of Excellence and the FDNY WTC Data Center, are in a unique position to study health outcomes, such as cancer, as we are able to estimate pre- and post-9/11 cancer rates in non–WTC exposed rescue workers, both those retired prior to and those hired after closure of the WTC site as a comparison for WTC-exposed workers. We are able to do this because we continue to follow virtually the entire WTC-exposed and non–WTC exposed cohorts through matches with various state cancer registries. Furthermore, by having two occupational groups (Fire and EMS) with well-documented but quite different exposures, we have high and low exposed groups for comparison studies. Inasmuch as FDNY Bureau of Health Services (BHS) cares for both these groups using the same surveillance protocols and each group has identical access to healthcare, comparisons of cancer rates between these groups should limit the potential for surveillance bias.

FDNY has developed a cancer database that collects and documents cases of cancer reported: 1) in the annual monitoring questionnaires; 2) in the FDNY electronic medical record during any treatment visit; and 3) via matches with state cancer registries. This has led to a nearly complete dataset for both pre- and post-9/11 cancers. In this study, follow-up began in 1996 because this is when cancer data from New York State Cancer Registry reached high levels of completeness (>97%).

We have just completed our first cancer study in this cohort—examining cancers occurring within the first seven years post-9/11/2001 in approximately 10,000 firefighters.

Additional research is needed as the time interval since 9/11 is still short for cancer outcome studies. As in any observational study, it is also challenging to rule out the effect of surveillance bias or potential unmeasured confounders. Furthermore, FDNY firefighters experienced uniquely intense WTC exposures and therefore our findings need to be reproduced in other groups with different but equally well-documented exposures and similar access to healthcare. Our FDNY EMS workers are a perfect group for this comparison analysis.

---

[8] Excerpted from a letter to John Howard submitted on June 21, 2011, by David Prezant, M.D., Chief Medical Officer and Special Advisor to the New York City Fire Commissioner on Health Policy, Principal Investigator, WTC Data Center, Co-Director FDNY WTC Medical Monitoring and Treatment Programs, and Kerry Kelly, M.D., Chief Medical Officer, Bureau of Health Services, FDNY, Principal Investigator, WTC Clinical Center of Excellence, Co-Director WTC Medical Monitoring and Treatment Programs.

To fund this additional research, we have recently submitted to NIOSH a research application that would allow us to continue our study of cancer rates of incident (first cancers) and multiple primary tumors, in separate cohorts of firefighters and EMS workers. This future research, if funded, will build upon the knowledge and analytic experience our team gained from this initial study by extending the study to include additional years of follow-up for firefighters, and for the first time, by studying our EMS population. Continuing this research by leveraging the existing infrastructure and the established trust that the FDNY clinical and data centers have built with this cohort will provide an effective path to reach this important scientific objective.

This research would benefit the WTC program and the cohort it serves. If cancer rates are increased, then a screening and treatment program can be tailored to the specific sites or organs that are affected and the cohort can receive targeted education on strategies to prevent and find new cancers. In contrast, if these analyses show that cancer is not increased in the two different groups (Fire and EMS) with well-documented but different exposures and similar access to healthcare (e.g., similar case surveillance issues), then this information can be communicated to the cohort in a responsible fashion, emphasizing that longer-term studies are needed, but that until there is evidence to the contrary, limited healthcare dollars should be directed otherwise.

2. Mount Sinai School of Medicine[9]

a. Any clinically observed findings, including trends, that are unpublished, but which you believe are important clinical observations pertaining to cancer?

In 2009, the World Trade Center Medical Monitoring and Treatment Program (WTC MMTP) published the manuscript "Multiple Myeloma in World Trade Center Responders." The study reported an unusual number of multiple myeloma cases in World Trade Center responders under age 45. As a case series, it did not permit the drawing of causal inference. Nonetheless, the report underscored the importance of maintaining surveillance for cancer and other emerging diseases in this highly exposed population.

Currently, we are actively investigating and analyzing almost 60 cancer sites, including myeloma, to determine if there is any evidence of elevation in rates. Preliminary data are undergoing detailed analysis and review by Dr. Paolo Boffetta, an expert in the field of cancer epidemiology, and by others.

b. Any planned data analysis or research efforts pertaining to cancer?

In June 2010, we participated in an expert meeting with the Fire Department of New York City, New York City Department of Health Registry, nationally

---

[9] Excerpted from a June 22, 2011, letter to John Howard submitted by Philip J. Landrigan, M.D., M.Sc., Ethel H. Wise Professor and Chairman, Department of Preventive Medicine, Professor of Pediatrics, Director, Environmental Health Center, and Principal Investigator of WTC Medical Monitoring and Treatment Program and WTC Data Center, Mount Sinai School of Medicine, New York, New York.

recognized biostatisticians, environmental health scientists and cancer epidemiologists to develop strategies and methods that may be utilized to analyze WTC data for cancer.

Currently, our focus of work is on the linkage of data from the WTC MMTP with data from the New York State Tumor Registry (and other State Tumor Registries as the data becomes available) in order to identify responders that have been diagnosed with cancer and who are also registered with New York State Tumor Registry. Analysis of data will involve a comparison of the number of cancer cases identified in State Tumor Registries among WTC responders with expected numbers of cancer in the general population (based on the responders' age, sex, and race).

Furthermore, the WTC MMTP Cancer Surveillance Team continues to work intensively to confirm all self-reported cancers. We have hired a senior, highly experienced nurse who is engaged in the process of interviewing every responder who has reported cancer. She is asking for permission to obtain these responders' medical records from hospitals and physicians so that all reported diagnoses of cancer can be properly verified and classified.

Additionally, we will utilize exposure data to determine whether responders with increased exposure are more likely to be diagnosed with cancer (and identified in the Tumor Registry). Our initial efforts will look at responders who were present at the WTC sites and in the dust cloud on 9/11. Also, we will look at duration of work at the WTC sites. In time, we will develop a more sophisticated exposure matrix that combines duration of work, presence on 9/11–12, and location and type of work.

c. Any findings pertaining to cancer that are being prepared by you for publication, with an estimate when such paper(s) are expected to be published?

At this time, we are preparing an application for the Department of Health and Human Services solicitation number 2011-Q-13340 for further surveillance, analysis and reporting on all cancers.

3. World Trade Center Health Registry[10]

The World Trade Center (WTC) Health Registry is in the early stages of analyzing any potential relationship between cancer and WTC exposure among its 71,000 enrollees. Because the induction period (the time it takes for cancers to develop) and the latency period (the time to detection) can range from five to 20 years after environmental or occupational exposures, this research will continue for as long as the Registry is funded.

---

[10] Information submitted to John Howard on June 20, 2011, via email by Mark Farfel, Sc.D., Director of the WTC Health Registry at the New York City Department of Health and Mental Hygiene.

Physicians are required by law to report information to state cancer registries about cancer diagnoses among their patients. As a first step in its cancer analysis, the WTC Health Registry is confirming cancer diagnoses by matching the names of its enrollees with cancer registries in New York and 10 other states where more than 90% of all enrollees currently reside. This is a critical step because it provides researchers with essential information, including the date of diagnosis and the type of cancer. This summer, the Registry expects to complete matches through 2008 in all 11 states (there is a lag between the time physicians report cancer data and when the state is able to compile it). Future matches will take place every 2 years.

Once the WTC Health Registry has completed the matches to all 11 state cancer registries through 2008, it will conduct a preliminary analysis of the data to determine if there is an excess incidence of post 9/11 cancer overall, and by specific types of cancer, among enrollees by comparing the number of cancer diagnoses among enrollees to those expected based on rates among the general population of New York State (the New York State Cancer Registry calculates the incidence of cancer based on gender, age and ethnicity). This is known as an external comparison.

The WTC Health Registry plans to submit the results of this first, or baseline, analysis among enrollees compared with New York State cancer rates for publication early in 2012. Thereafter, the WTC Health Registry plans to conduct similar analyses every five years, using matches from all 11 state cancer registries and comparing them to rates of cancer in New York State because the Registry population is believed to be most similar to that of New York State. External comparisons may also be made to the general U.S. population. This will facilitate comparison of findings with WTC researchers who may be using this population for their analyses.

In addition, the WTC Health Registry will attempt to conduct internal comparisons based on the degree (high, intermediate, low) to which an enrollee was exposed to the WTC disaster. A group of national experts, including representatives from the American Cancer Society, Memorial Sloane Kettering Hospital and Harvard University, recommended that WTC cancer researchers use internal comparisons whenever possible because they are likely to have greater scientific validity than external comparisons. However, internal comparisons are challenging for two reasons: 1) even though the Registry has the largest cohort of persons exposed to 9/11, the cohort is relatively small, thus limiting the statistical power of cancer analyses; and 2) information about specific types of WTC exposure is limited.

The WTC Health Registry is committed to employing the best methodology possible in its ongoing investigation to determine any potential links between WTC exposure and increased cancer risk. As part of this commitment, it will continue to work with other WTC researchers, including those from the Fire Department of New York and the New York/New Jersey WTC Clinical Consortium, in the WTC Analytic Methods

Workgroup, which was established to implement the recommendations from national experts in June 2010. These recommendations can be accessed in the 2010 WTC Medical Working Group's Annual Report.[11] In addition, the WTC Health Registry will continue to consult with these and other experts, as needed.

D. New York State Department of Health[12]

The WTC Responders Fatality Investigation (RFI) program was the data collection center for fatalities occurring among the WTC responder, worker and volunteer populations in order to conduct an initial assessment regarding whether responders were at high risk for certain causes of death. The study population included any responder death that occurred between September 12, 2001 and June 30, 2009. Because there was no central method to identify the responders, deaths were identified primarily through obituary reviews and names provided by other WTC programs.

A sample cohort was created using information from the WTC Health Registry. There were 836 deaths identified; the cause of death was confirmed for 814 deaths. Capture-recapture analyses indicated approximately 53% of expected deaths were identified. Because the ascertainment of deaths was incomplete, it was determined that the results of the PMRs were biased and unreliable. Few of the SMRs were elevated or statistically significant, primarily due to the healthy worker effect and low case ascertainment.

Because the results of this study were inconclusive, it is recommended that the currently established WTC programs conduct death matching of their cohorts on a periodic basis to examine whether there is an increased risk among their cohorts. Elevated results should be used to generate hypotheses for future research.

---

[11] 2010 WTC Medical Working Group's Annual Report can be found at http://www.nyc.gov/html/doh/wtc/downloads/pdf/news/2010_mwg_annual_report.pdf.

[12] Submitted to John Howard via email on June 20, 2011, by Kitty H. Gelberg, Ph.D., M.P.H., Chief, Epidemiology and Surveillance Section, Bureau of Occupational Health, New York State Department of Health, Troy, New York.

VI. Discussion of Findings

A. Exposure Publications

Following the September 11, 2001, terrorist attacks, environmental sampling of the area around the WTC in New York City identified 287 chemicals and chemical groups. Categories of these chemicals include asbestos and glass fibers, crystalline silica, various metals, volatile organic compounds, polychlorinated polycyclic compounds, and polycyclic aromatic hydrocarbons. Some of the chemicals identified through environmental sampling are known to be human carcinogens or are reasonably anticipated to be human carcinogens. These known or reasonably anticipated human carcinogens have been associated by the IARC and/or the NTP with a number of different types of cancers, such as lung cancer including mesothelioma; skin cancer; bladder cancer; hematopoietic cancers; testicular cancer; prostate cancer; and liver and biliary cancer.

A number of exposure assessments were conducted within the first few months after the September 11, 2001, terrorist attacks and published in the scientific and medical literature. The peer-reviewed, published assessments suggest that responders and others in the nearby area were potentially exposed to one or more of the substances designated by IARC and NTP as known or reasonably anticipated human carcinogens, although generally not in excess of applicable occupational exposure limits.

A significant limitation of the exposure assessment literature is the paucity of personal exposure measurements, especially during the early stage of the September 11th disaster when exposures were the most intense. These limitations in the exposure assessment literature make scientific analysis of a causal association between exposure and health effects, such as cancer, quite challenging. Furthermore, the science of conducting risk assessments of complex mixed exposures, such as those that occurred as a result of the September 11, 2001, terrorist attacks, adds another dimension to the challenge.

B. Cancer Publications

Very little has been published addressing the association of exposures arising from the September 11, 2001, terrorist attacks and cancer in responders and survivors. Only one peer-reviewed article (on any type of cancer) has been published to date [Moline 2009]. Two other publications used models to estimate the risk of cancer among residents in Lower Manhattan, with one noting a "slightly elevated" risk of cancer [Rayne 2005] and another finding a "negligible" risk of cancer associated with assumed exposure to asbestos [Nolan et al. 2005]. The paucity of published epidemiologic studies on cancer in the peer-reviewed literature to date may be due to a number of factors, including the traditional latency period between exposure and the development of cancer. However, human health research in the area of cancer associated with the September 11, 2001, terrorist attacks is ongoing, and peer-reviewed publications will be included in future periodic reviews of cancer.

C. Determination

The first periodic review of cancer for the WTC Health Program provides a summary of the current scientific and medical findings in the peer-reviewed literature about exposures resulting from the September 11, 2001, terrorist attacks and cancer studies. The review discusses criteria that have been used previously to assist in weighing the evidence to determine if a causal association exists between exposure and cancer. The review summarizes input from the public and provides reports about cancer from the Mount Sinai School of Medicine, Bureau of Health Services of FDNY, the WTC Health Registry of the New York City Department of Health and Mental Hygiene, and the New York State Department of Health.

Based on the scientific and medical findings in the peer-reviewed literature reported in this first periodic review of cancer for the WTC Health Program, insufficient evidence exists at this time to propose a rule to add cancer, or a certain type of cancer, to the List of WTC-Related Health Conditions.

Although a determination cannot be made to propose a rule to add cancer, or a type of cancer, to the List of WTC-Related Health Conditions at this time, it is important to point out that the current absence of published scientific and medical findings demonstrating a causal association between the exposures resulting from the September 11, 2001, terrorist attacks and the occurrence of cancer in responders and survivors does not indicate evidence of the absence of a causal association.

It is expected that the second periodic review of cancer for the WTC Health Program will be conducted in early to mid-2012 to capture any emerging findings about exposures and cancer in responders and survivors affected by the September 11, 2001, terrorist attacks.

It is hoped that the findings from the first periodic review of cancer will assist the WTC Health Program Scientific/Technical Advisory Committee in its responsibility to review scientific and medical evidence and to make advisory recommendations to the Administrator about adding health conditions to the List of WTC-Related Health Conditions.

Appendix A. References

ACS (American Cancer Society) [2010]. Cancer facts and figures 2010. [http://www.cancer.org/acs/groups/content/@epidemiologysurveilance/documents/document/acspc-026238.pdf]. Date accessed: June 14, 2011.

Breysse PN, Williams DL, Herbstman JB, Symons JM, Chillrud SN, Ross J, Henshaw S, Res K, Watson M, Geyh A [2005]. Asgestos exposures to truck drivers during World Trade Center cleanup operations. J Occ Env Health 2:400–405.

Butt CM, Diamond ML, Truong J, Ikonomou MG, Helm PA, Stern GA [2004]. Semivolatile organic compounds in window films from lower Manhattan after the September 11th World Trade Center attacks. Environ Sci Technol 38:3514–3524.

Calderoni ME, Alderman EM, Silver EJ, Bauman LJ [2006]. The mental health impact of 9/11 on inner-city high school students 20 miles north of Ground Zero. Journal of Adolescent Health 39(1):57–65.

Clark R, Green R, Swayze G, Swayze GA, Meeker G, Sutley S, Hoefen TM, Livo KE, Plumlee G, Pavri B, Sarture C, Wilson S, Hageman P, Lamothe P, Vance JS, Boardman J, Brownfield I, Gent C, Morath LC, Taggart J, Theodorakos PM, Adams M [2001]. Environmental studies of the World Trade Center area after the September 11, 2001 attack. U.S. Geological Survey Open-File Report 01-0429. [http://pubs.usgs.gov/of/2001/ofr-01-0429/]. Date accessed: June 14, 2011.

COPC Committee (Contaminants of Potential Concern) [2003]. World Trade Center indoor environment assessment: selecting contaminants of potential concern and setting health-based benchmarks. [http://epa.gov/WTC/reports/contaminants_of_concern_benchmark_study.pdf]. Date accessed: June 14, 2011.

DiGrande L, Perrin MA, Thorpe LE, Thajli L, Murphy J, Wu D, Farfel M, Brackbill RM [2008]. Posttraumatic stress symptoms, PTSD, and risk factors among Lower Manhattan residents 2–3 years after the September 11, 2001 terrorist attacks. Journal Traumatic Stress 21(3):264–273.

DiGrande L, Neria Y, Brackbill RM, Pulliam P, Galea S [2011]. Long-term posttraumatic stress symptoms among 3,271 civilian survivors of the September 11, 2001, terrorist attacks on the World Trade Center. Am J Epidemiol 173(3):271–281.

Doll R [2002]. Proof of causality: deduction from epidemiological observation. Perspect Bio Med 45:499–515.

Driscoll T, Nelson DI, Steenland K, Leigh J, Concha-Barrientos M, Fingerhut M [2005]. The global burden of disease due to occupational carcinogens. Am J Ind Med 48(6):419–431.

Eaton DL, Klaassen CD [1999]. Principles of toxicology. In Klaassen CD, Watkins III JB, eds. Casarett and Doull's toxicology: the basic science of poisons. 5th ed. New York: McGraw-Hill Companies, Inc.

Edelman P, Osterloh J, Pirkle J, Caudill SP, Grainger J, Jones R, Blunt B, Calafat A, Turner W, Feldman D, Baron S, Bernard B, Lushniak BD, Kelly K, Prezant D [2003]. Biomonitoring of chemical exposure among New York City firefighters responding to the World Trade Center fire and collapse. Environ Health Perspect *111*:1906–1911.

Endara SM, Ryan MAK, Sevick CJ, Conlin AMS, Macera CA, Smith TC [2009]. Does acute maternal stress in pregnancy affect infant health outcomes? Examination of a large cohort of infants born after the terrorist attacks of September 11, 2001. BMC Public Health 9:252.

Feldman DM, Baron SL, Bernard BP, Lushniak BD, Banauch G, Arcentales N, Kelly KJ, Prezant DJ [2004]. Symptoms, respirator use, and pulmonary function changes among New York City firefighters responding to the World Trade Center disaster. Chest *125*(4):1256–1264.

Fireman EM, Lerman Y, Ganor E, Greif J, Fireman-Shoresh S, Lioy PJ, Banauch GI, Weiden M, Kelly KJ, Prezant DJ [2004]. Induced sputum assessment in New York City firefighters exposed to World Trade Center dust. Environ Health Perspect *112*:1564–1569.

Fitzgerald SD, Rumbeiha WK, Emmett Braselton W, Downend AB, Otto CM [2008]. Pathology and toxicology findings for search-and-rescue dogs deployed to the September 11, 2001, terrorist attack sites: initial five-year surveillance. J Vet Diagn Invest *20*(4):477–484.

Fox PR, Puschner B, Ebel JG [2008]. Assessment of acute injuries, exposure to environmental toxins, and five-year health surveillance of New York Police Department working dogs following the September 11, 2001, World Trade Center terrorist attack. J Am Vet Med Assoc *233*(1):48–59.

Galea S, Vlahov D, Resnick H, Ahern J, Susser E, Gold J, Bucuvalas M, Kilpatrick D [2003]. Trends of probable post-traumatic stress disorder in New York City after the September 11 terrorist attacks. Am J Epidemiol *158*(6):514–524.

Gavett SH, Haykal-Coates N, Highfill JW, Ledgbetter AD, Chen LC, Cohen MD, Harkema JR, Wagner JG, Costa DL [2003]. "World Trade Center fine particulate matter causes respiratory tract hyperresponsiveness in mice." Environ Health Perspect *111*(7):981–991.

Geyh AS, Chillrud S, Williams DL, Herbstman J, Symons JM, Rees K, Ross J, Kim SR, Lim HJ, Turpin B, Breysse P [2005]. Assessing truck driver exposure at the World Trade Center disaster site: personal and area monitoring for particulate matter and volatile organic compounds during October 2001 and April 2002. J Occup Environ Hyg *2*(3):179–193.

Herdt-Losavio ML [2008]. Development of an exposure assessment method for epidemiological studies of New York State pesonnel who responded to the WTC disaster. Ann Occup Hyg 2008; *52*:83–93.

Hill AB [1965]. The environment and disease: Association or causation? Proc R Soc Med *58*:295–300.

Horii Y, Jiang Q, Hanari N, Lam PK, Yamashita N, Jansing R, Aldous KM, Mauer MP, Eadon GA, Kannan K [2010]. Polychlorinated dibenzo-p-dioxins, dibenzofurans, biphenyls, and naphthalenes in plasma of workers deployed at the World Trade Center after the collapse. Environ Sci Technol *44*(13):5188–5194.

IARC (International Agency for Research on Cancer, World Health Organization) [2006]. IARC monographs on the evaluation of carcinogenic risks to humans: preamble. Lyon, France, 2006.

IOM (Institute of Medicine) [2009]. Veterans and Agent Orange: Update 2008. Washington, DC: The National Academies Press.

IOM (Institute of Medicine) [2010]. Health effects of serving in the Gulf War Update 2009. Washington, DC: The National Academies Press.

Landrigan PJ, Lioy PJ, Thurston G, Berkowitz G, Chen LC, Chillrud SN, Gavett SH, Georgopoulos PG, Geyh AS, Levin S, Perera F, Rappaport SM, Small C [2004]. Health and environmental consequences of the world trade center disaster. Environ Health Perspect *112*(6):731–739.

Landrigan PJ, Forman J, Galvez M, Newman B, Engel SM, Chemtob C [2008]. Impact of September 11 World Trade Center disaster on children and pregnant women. Mt Sinai J Med *75*:129–134.

Lederman SA, Jones RL, Caldwell KL, Rauh V, Sheets SE, Tang D, Viswanathan S, Becker M, Stein JL, Wang RY, Perera FP [2008]. Relation between cord blood mercury levels and early child development in a World Trade Center cohort. Environ Health Perspect *116*(8):1085–1091.

Lemen R [2004]. Chrysotile asbestos as a cause of mesothelioma. Int J Occup Environ Health *10*:233–239.

Lioy PJ, Gochfeld M [2002]. Lessons learned on environmental, occupational, and residential exposures from the attack on the World Trade Center. Am J Ind Med *42*(6):560–565.

Lioy PJ, Georgopoulos P [2006]. The anatomy of the exposures that occurred around the World Trade Center site: 9/11 and beyond. Ann N Y Acad Sci *1076*:54–79.

Litten S, McChesney DJ, Hamilton MC, Fowler B [2003]. Destruction of the World Trade Center and PCBs, PBDEs, PCDD/Fs, PBDD/Fs, and chlorinated biphenylenes in water, sediment, and sewage sludge. Environ Sci Technol 37(24):5502–5510.

Lorber M [2003]. Assessment of dioxin inhalation exposures and potential health impacts following the collapse of the World Trade Center Towers. Organohalogen Compounds, 63, 324–327.

Lorber M, Gibb H, Grant L, Pinto J, Pleil J, Cleverly D [2007] Assessment of inhalation exposures and potential health risks to the general population that resulted from the collapse of the World Trade Center towers. Risk Anal 27(5):1203–21.

Lucas RM, McMichael AJ [2005]. Association of causation: evaluating links between "environment and disease." Bulletin of the World Health Organization 85(10):792–795.

Marinaccio A, Binazzi A, Marzio DD, Scarselli A, Verardo M, Mirabelli D, Gennaro V, Mensi C, Riboldi L, Merler E, De Zotti R, Romanelli A, Chellini E, Silvestri S, Pascucci C, Romeo E, Menegozzo S, Musti M, Cavone D, Cauzillo G, Tumino R, Nicita C, Melis M, Iavicoli S [2011]. Pleural malignant mesothelioma epidemic. Incidence, modalities of asbestos exposure and occupations involved from the Italian national register. Int J Cancer. 2011 Jun 6. doi: 10.1002/ijc.26229.

McGee JK, Chen LC, Cohen MD, Chee GR, Prophete CM, Haykal-Coates N, Wasson SJ, Conner TL, Costa DL, Gavett SH [2003]. Chemical analysis of World Trade Center fine particulate matter for use in toxicologic assessment. Environ Health Perspect 111(7):972–980.

Miller A [2009]. World Trade Center multiple myeloma: police responders only? J Occup Environ Med 51(12):1357; author reply 1357–1358.

Moline J, Herbert R, Nguyen N [2006]. Health consequences of the September 11 World Trade Center attacks: a review. Cancer Invest 24(3):294–301.

Moline JM, Herbert R, Crowley L, Troy K, Hodgman E, Shukla G, Udasin I, Luft B, Wallenstein S, Landrigan P, Savitz DA [2009a]. Multiple myeloma in World Trade Center responders: a case series. J Occup Environ Med 51(8):896–902.

Moline JM, Herbert R, Crowley L, Troy K, Hodgman E, Shukla G, Udasin I, Luft B, Wallenstein S, Landrigan P, Savitz DA [2009b]. World Trade Center Multiple Myeloma: Police Responders Only? Response. J Occup Environ Med 51(12):1357–1358.

Neria Y, Olfson M, Gameroff MJ, DiGrande L, Wickramaratne P, Gross R, Pilowsky D, Neugebaur R et al. [2010]. Long-term course of probably PTSD after the 9/11 attacks: A study in urban primary care. Journal Traumatic Stress 23(4):474–482.

Nicholson WJ, Rohl AN, Ferrand EF [1971]. Asbestos air pollution in New York City. In Proceedings of the Second Clean Air Congress. New York, Academic Press, pp. 36–139.

Nolan RP, Ross M, Nord GL, Axten CW, Osleeb JP, Domnin SG, Price B, Wilson R. [2005]. Risk assessment for asbestos-related cancer from the 9/11 attack on the World Trade Center. J Occup Environ Med 8:817–825.

NIOSH [1994a]. Method 7400 'Asbestos and Other Fibers by PCM', Issue 2 (8/15/94). In: NIOSH Manual of Analytical Methods (Fourth Edition). National Institute for Occupational Safety and Health, Cincinnati, OH, DHHS (NIOSH) Publication No. 2003-154. [http://www.cdc.gov/niosh/nmam/pdfs/7400.pdf]. Date accessed: June 30, 2008.

NIOSH [1994b]. Method 7402 'Asbestos by TEM', Issue 2 (8/15/94). In: NIOSH Manual of Analytical Methods (Fourth Edition). National Institute for Occupational Safety and Health, Cincinnati, OH, DHHS (NIOSH) Publication No. 2003-154. [http://www.cdc.gov/niosh/nmam/pdfs/7402.pdf]. Date accessed: June 30, 2008.

NRC (National Research Council) [2009]. Science and decisions: advancing risk assessment. Washington, DC: National Academies Press.

NTP (National Toxicology Program) [2011]. 12th Report on Carcinogens. National Toxicology Program, Public Health Service, U.S. Department of Health and Human Services, Research Triangle Park, NC. [http://ntp-server.niehs.nih]. Date accessed: June 14, 2011.

Offenberg JH, Eisenreich SJ, Chen LC, Cohen MD, Chee G, Prophete C, Weisel C, Lioy PJ [2004]. Persistent organic pollutants in the dusts that settled across lower Manhattan after September 11, 2001. Environ Sci Technol 37:502–508.

Olson DA, Norris GA, Landis MS, Vette AF [2004]. Chemical characterization of ambient particulate matter near the World Trade Center: elemental carbon, organic carbon, and mass reconstruction. Environ Sci Technol 38:4465–4473.

Osinubi OYO, Gandhi SK, Ohman-Strickland P, Boglarsky C, Fiedler N, Kipen H, Robson M [2008]. Organizational factors and office workers' health after the World Trade Center terrorist attacks: Long-term physical symptoms, psychological distress, and work productivity. J Occup Environ Med 50(2):112–125.

Otto CM, Downend AB, Moore GE, Daggy JK, Ranivand DL, Reetz JA, Fitzgerald SD [2010]. Medical surveillance of search dogs deployed to the World Trade Center and Pentagon: 2001–2006. J Environ Health 73(2):12–21.

Otto CM, Downend AB, Serpell JA, Ziemer LS, Saunders HM [2004]. Medical and behavioral surveillance of dogs deployed to the World Trade Center and the Pentagon from October 2001 to June 2002. J Am Vet Med Assoc 225(6):861–867.

Payne JP, Kemp SJ, Dewar A, Goldstraw P, Kendall M, Chen LC, Tetley TD [2004]. Effects of Airborne World Trade Center Dust on Cytokine Release by Primary Human Lung Cells In Vitro. J Occup Environ Med 46(5):420–427.

Parekh P, Semkow TM, Husain L, Wozniak GJ [2002]. Tritium in the World Trade Center Disaster: Its possible sources and fate. Abstr Pap Am Chem Soc 223:026-NUCL.

Perera FP, Tang D, Whyatt R, Lederman SA, Jedrychowski W [2005a]. DNA damage from polycyclic aromatic hydrocarbons measured by benzo[a]pyrene-DNA adducts in mothers and newborns from Northern Manhattan, the World Trade Center Area, Poland, and China. Cancer Epidemiol Biomarkers Prev 14(3):709–714.

Perera FP, Tang D, Rauh V, Lester K, Tsai WY, Tu YH, Weiss L, Hoepner L, King J, Del Priore G, Lederman SA [2005b]. Relationships among polycyclic aromatic hydrocarbon-DNA adducts, proximity to the World Trade Center, and effects on fetal growth. Environ Health Perspect 113(8):1062–1067.

Perera FP, Tang D, Rauh V, Tu YH, Tsai WY, Becker M, Stein JL, King J, Del Priore G, Lederman SA [2007]. Relationship between polycyclic aromatic hydrocarbon-DNA adducts, environmental tobacco smoke, and child development in the World Trade Center cohort. Environ Health Perspect 115(10):1497–1502.

Pleil JD, Vette AF, Johnson BA, Rappaport SM [2004]. Air levels of carcinogenic polycyclic aromatic hydrocarbons after the World Trade Center disaster. Proc Natl Acad Sci U S A. 101:11685–11688.

Pleil JD, Lorber MN [2007]. Relative congener scaling of Polychlorinated dibenzo-p-dioxins and dibenzofurans to estimate building fire contributions in air, surface wipes, and dust samples. Environ Sci Technol 41:7286–7293.

Rayne S [2005]. Using exterior building surface films to assess human exposure and health risks from PCDD/Fs in New York City, USA, after the World Trade Center attacks. J Hazard Mater 127:33–39.

Rayne S, Ikonomou MG, Butt CM, Diamond ML, Truong J [2005]. Polychlorinated dioxins and furans from the World Trade Center attacks in exterior window films from lower Manhattan in New York City. Environ Sci Technol 39:1995–2003.

Reibman J, Lin S, Hwang SA, et al. [2005] The World Trade Center resident's respiratory health study: New-onset respiratory symptoms and pulmonary function. Environ Health Perspect 113:406–411.

Rom WN, Weiden M, Garcia R, Ting AY, Vathesatogkit P, Tse DB, McGuinness G, Roggli V, Prezant D [2002]. Acute eosinophilic pneumonia in a New York City firefighter exposed to World Trade Center dust. American Journal of Respiratory and Critical Care Medicine 166(6):797–800.

Rothman KJ, Greenland S [1998]. Modern epidemiology, 2nd ed. Philadelphia: Lippencott-Raven Publishers.

Rothman KJ [2008]. Epidemiology: An introduction. Oxford University Press, USA.

Rosati JA, Bern AM, Willis RD, Blanchard FT, Conner TL, Kahn HD, Friedman D [2004]. September 11th World Trade Center attacks. Environ Sci Technol 38:3514–3524.

Semkow TM, Hafner RS, Parekh PP, Wozniak GJ, Haines DK, Husain L, Rabun RL, Williams PG [2002]. Elevated tritium levels at the World Trade Center. [http://www.escholarship.org/uc/item/4xq88667]. Date accessed 06/25/2011.

Slensky KA, Drobatz KJ, Downend AB, Otto CM [2004]. Deployment morbidity among search-and-rescue dogs used after the September 11, 2001, terrorist attacks. J Am Vet Med Assoc 225(6):868–873.

Skloot G, Goldman M, Fischler D, Goldman C, Schechter C, Levin S, Teirstein A [2004]. Respiratory symptoms and physiologic assessment of ironworkers at the World Trade Center disaster site. Chest 125(4):1248–1255.

Swartz E, Stockburger L, Vallero DA [2003]. Polycyclic aromatic hydrocarbons and other semivolatile organic compounds collected in New York City in response to the events of 9/11. Environ Sci Technol 37:3537–3546.

Tao L, Kannan K, Aldous KM, Mauer MP, Eadon GA [2008]. Biomonitoring of perfluorochemicals in plasma of New York State personnel responding to the World Trade Center disaster. Environ Sci Technol 42:3472–3478.

Wallingford KM, Snyder EM [2001]. Occupational exposures during the World Trade Center disaster response. Toxicol Ind Health 17:247–253.

Wang S, Prophete C, Soukup JM, Chen LC, Costa M, Ghio A, Qu QS, Cohen MD, Chen HB [2010]. Roles of MAPK pathway activation during cytokine induction in BEAS-2B cells exposed to fine World Trade Center (WTC) dust. J Immunotoxicol 7(4):298–307.

Weed DL [2005]. Weight of evidence: A review of concept and methods. Risk Analysis 25(6):1545–1557.

Wolff MS, Teitelbaum SL, Lioy PJ, Santella RM, Wang RY, Jones RL, Caldwell KL, Sjodin A, Turner WE, Li W, Georgopoulos P, Berkowitz G [2005]. Exposures among pregnant women near the World Trade Center site on 9/11. Environ Health Perspect 113:739–748.

Wolff MS, Teitelbaum SL, Lioy PJ, Santella RM, Wang RY, Jones RL, Caldwell KL, Sjodin A, Turner WE, Li W, Georgopoulos P, Berkowitz G [2005]. Exposures among pregnant women near the World Trade Center site on 11 September 2001. Environ Health Perspect 113:739–748.

Wu M, Gordon RE, Herbert R Padilla M, Moline J, Mendelson D, Litle V, Travis WD, Gil J [2010]. Case report: Lung disease in World Trade Center responders exposed to dust and smoke: carbon nanotubes found in the lungs of World Trade Center patients and dust samples. Environ Health Perspect 118:499–504.

Yiin LM, Millette JR, Vette A, Ilacqua, V, Quan C, Gorczynski J, Kendall M, Lung CC, Welsel CP, Ill Y, Buckley BI, Lioy PJ [2004]. Comparisons of the dust/smoke particulate that settled inside the surrounding buildings and outside on the streets of southern New York City after the collapse of the World Trade Center, September 11, 2001. J Air Waste Manag Assoc 54(5):515–528.

Appendix B. Exposure Publications

A. Peer-Reviewed

Adams RE, Boscarino JA [2005]. Stress and well-being in the aftermath of the World Trade Center attack: The continuing effects of a communitywide disaster. J Community Psychol 33(2):175–190.

Adams RE, Boscarino JA, Galea S [2006]. Social and psychological resources and health outcomes after the World Trade Center disaster. Soc Sci Med 62(1):176–188.

Agronick G, Stueve A, Vargo S, O'Donnell L [2007]. New York City young adults' psychological reactions to 9/11: findings from the Reach for Health longitudinal study. Am J Community Psychol 39(1–2):79–90.

Aldrich TK, Gustave J, Hall CB, Cohen HW, Webber MP, Zeig-Owens R, Cosenza K, Christodoulou V, Glass L, Al-Othman F, Weiden MD, Kelly KJ, Prezant DJ [2010]. Lung function in rescue workers at the World Trade Center after 7 years. N Engl J Med 362(14):1263–1272.

Allegra JR, Mostashari F, Rothman J, Milano P, Cochrane DG [2005]. Cardiac events in New Jersey after the September 11, 2001, terrorist attack. J Urban Health 82(3):358–363.

Allshouse WB, Pleil JD, Rappaport SM, Serre ML [2009]. Mass fraction spatiotemporal geostatistics and its application to map atmospheric polycyclic aromatic hydrocarbons after 9/11. Stoch Env Res Risk A 23(8):1213–1223.

Altman KW, Desai SC, Moline J, de la Hoz RE, Herbert R, Gannon PJ, Doty RL [2011]. Odor identification ability and self-reported upper respiratory symptoms in workers at the post-9/11 World Trade Center site. Int Arch Occup Environ Health 84(2):131–137.

Banauch GI, Alleyne D, Sanchez R, Olender K, Cohen HW, Weiden M, Kelly KJ, Prezant DJ [2003]. Persistent hyperreactivity and reactive airway dysfunction in firefighters at the World Trade Center. Am J Respir Crit Care Med 168(1):54–62.

Banauch GI, Brantly M, Izbicki G, Hall C, Shanske A, Chavko R, Santhyadka G, Christodoulou V, Weiden MD, Prezant DJ [2010]. Accelerated spirometric decline in New York City firefighters with alpha-antitrypsin deficiency. Chest 138(5):1116–1124.

Banauch GI, Dhala A, Alleyne D, Alva R, Santhyadka G, Krasko A, Weiden M, Kelly KJ, Prezant DJ [2005]. Bronchial hyperreactivity and other inhalation lung injuries in rescue/recovery workers after the World Trade Center collapse. Crit Care Med 33(1 Suppl):S102–106.

Banauch GI, Hall C, Weiden M, Cohen HW, Aldrich TK, Christodoulou V, Arcentales N, Kelly KJ, Prezant DJ [2006]. Pulmonary function after exposure to the World Trade

Center collapse in the New York City Fire Department. Am J Respir Crit Care Med *174*(3):312–319.

Berninger A, Webber MP, Cohen HW, Gustave J, Lee R, Niles JK, Chiu S, Zeig Owens R, Soo J, Kelly K, Prezant DJ [2010]. Trends of elevated PTSD risk in firefighters exposed to the World Trade Center disaster: 2001–2005. Public Health Rep *125*(4):556–566.

Berninger A, Webber MP, Niles JK, Gustave J, Lee R, Cohen HW, Kelly K, Corrigan M, Prezant DJ [2010]. Longitudinal study of probable post-traumatic stress disorder in firefighters exposed to the World Trade Center disaster. Am J Ind Med *53*(12):1177–1185.

Berninger A, Webber MP, Weakley J, Gustave J, Zeig-Owens R, Lee R, Al-Othman F, Cohen HW, Kelly K, Prezant DJ [2010]. Quality of life in relation to upper and lower respiratory conditions among retired 9/11-exposed firefighters with pulmonary disability. Qual Life Res *19*(10):1467–1476.

Berrios-Torres SI, Greenko JA, Phillips M, Miller JR, Treadwell T, Ikeda RM [2003]. World Trade Center rescue worker injury and illness surveillance, New York, 2001. Am J Prev Med *25*(2):79–87.

Bills CB, Dodson N, Stellman JM, Southwick S, Sharma V, Herbert R, Moline JM, Katz CL [2009]. Stories behind the symptoms: A qualitative analysis of the narratives of 9/11 rescue and recovery workers. Psychiatr Q *80*(3):173–189.

Bills CB, Levy NA, Sharma V, Charney DS, Herbert R, Moline J, Katz CL [2008]. Mental health of workers and volunteers responding to events of 9/11: review of the literature. Mt Sinai J Med *75*(2):115–127.

Boscarino JA, Galea S, Adams RE, Ahern J, Resnick H, Vlahov D [2004]. Mental health service and medication use in New York City after the September 11, 2001, terrorist attack. Psychiatr Serv *55*(3):274–283.

Bowers B, Hasni S, Gruber BL [2010]. Sarcoidosis in World Trade Center rescue workers presenting with rheumatologic manifestations. J Clin Rheumatol *16*(1):26–27.

Bowler RM, Han H, Gocheva V, Nakagawa S, Alper H, DiGrande L, Cone JE [2010]. Gender differences in probable posttraumatic stress disorder among police responders to the 2001 World Trade Center terrorist attack. Am J Ind Med *53*(12):1186–1196.

Brackbill RM, Hadler JL, DiGrande L, Ekenga CC, Farfel MR, Friedman S, Perlman SE, Stellman SD, Walker DJ, Wu D, Yu S, Thorpe LE [2009]. Asthma and posttraumatic stress symptoms 5 to 6 years following exposure to the World Trade Center terrorist attack. JAMA *302*(5):502–516.

Breysse PN, Williams DL, Herbstman JB, Symons JM, Chillrud SN, Ross J, Henshaw S, Rees K, Watson M, Geyh AS [2005]. Asbestos exposures to truck drivers during World Trade Center cleanup operations. J Occup Environ Hyg *2*(8):400–405.

Butt CM, Diamond ML, Truong J, Ikonomou MG, Helm PA, Stern GA [2004]. Semivolatile organic compounds in window films from lower Manhattan after the September 11th World Trade Center attacks. Environ Sci Technol 38(13):3514–3524.

Buyantseva LV, Tulchinsky M, Kapalka GM, Chinchilli VM, Qian Z, Gillio R, Roberts A, Bascom R [2007]. Evolution of lower respiratory symptoms in New York police officers after 9/11: a prospective longitudinal study. J Occup Environ Med 49(3):310–317.

Cahill TA, Cliff SS, Perry KD, Jimenez-Cruz M, Bench G, Grant P, Ueda D, Shackelford JF, Dunlap M, Meier M, Kelly PB, Riddle S, Selco J, Leifer R [2004]. Analysis of aerosols from the World Trade Center collapse site, New York, October 2 to October 30, 2001. Aerosol Sci Technol 38(2):165–183.

Calderoni ME, Alderman EM, Silver EJ, Bauman LJ [2006]. The mental health impact of 9/11 on inner-city high school students 20 miles north of Ground Zero. J Adolesc Health 39(1):57–65.

Chandran SK, Hawkshaw MJ, Sataloff RT [2009]. Otolaryngologic symptoms in persons exposed to World Trade Center dust and particle pollutants: a case for caution in declaring a diagnosis of WTC syndrome. Ear Nose Throat J 88(8):1067–1073.

Chen LC, Thurston G [2002]. World Trade Center cough. Lancet 360 Suppl:S37–38.

Chiu S, Niles JK, Webber MP, Zeig-Owens R, Gustave J, Lee R, Rizzotto L, Kelly KJ, Cohen HW, Prezant DJ [2011]. Evaluating Risk Factors and Possible Mediation Effects in Posttraumatic Depression and Posttraumatic Stress Disorder Comorbidity. Public Health Rep 126(2):201–209.

Cohen BS, Heikkinen MSA, Hazi Y [2004]. Airborne fine and ultrafine particles near the World Trade Center disaster site. Aerosol Sci Technol 38(4):338–348.

Colarossi L, Heyman J, Phillips M [2005]. Social workers' experiences of the World Trade Center disaster: Stressors and their relationship to symptom types. Community Ment Health J 41(2):185–198.

Crowley LE, Herbert R, Moline JM, Wallenstein S, Shukla G, Schechter C, Skloot GS, Udasin I, Luft BJ, Harrison D, Shapiro M, Wong K, Sacks HS, Landrigan PJ, Teirstein AS [2011]. "Sarcoid like" granulomatous pulmonary disease in World Trade Center disaster responders. Am J Ind Med 54(3):175–184.

Dahlgren J, Cecchini M, Takhar H, Paepke O [2007]. Persistent organic pollutants in 9/11 world trade center rescue workers: reduction following detoxification. Chemosphere 69(8):1320–1325.

Dalton PH, Opiekun RE, Gould M, McDermott R, Wilson T, Maute C, Ozdener MH, Zhao K, Emmett E, Lees PS, Herbert R, Moline J [2010]. Chemosensory loss: functional consequences of the world trade center disaster. Environ Health Perspect 118(9):1251–1256.

de Bocanegra HT, Moskalenko S, Chan P [2005]. PTSD and depression among displaced Chinese workers after the World Trade Center Attack: A follow-up study. J Urban Health 82(3):364–369.

de la Hoz RE, Aurora RN, Landsbergis P, Bienenfeld LA, Afilaka AA, Herbert R [2010]. Snoring and obstructive sleep apnea among former World Trade Center rescue workers and volunteers. J Occup Environ Med 52(1):29–32.

de la Hoz RE, Christie J, Teamer JA, Bienenfeld LA, Afilaka AA, Crane M, Levin SM, Herbert R [2008]. Reflux symptoms and disorders and pulmonary disease in former World Trade Center rescue and recovery workers and volunteers. J Occup Environ Med 50(12):1351–1354.

de la Hoz RE, Shohet MR, Bienenfeld LA, Afilaka AA, Levin SM, Herbert R [2008]. Vocal cord dysfunction in former World Trade Center (WTC) rescue and recovery workers and volunteers. Am J Ind Med 51(3):161–165.

de la Hoz RE, Shohet MR, Chasan R, Bienenfeld LA, Afilaka AA, Levin SM, Herbert R [2008]. Occupational toxicant inhalation injury: the World Trade Center (WTC) experience. Int Arch Occup Environ Health 81(4):479–485.

de la Hoz RE, Shohet MR, Wisnivesky JP, Bienenfeld LA, Afilaka AA, Herbert R [2009]. Atopy and upper and lower airway disease among former World Trade Center workers and volunteers. J Occup Environ Med 51(9):992–995.

DiGrande L, Neria Y, Brackbill RM, Pulliam P, Galea S [2011]. Long-term posttraumatic stress symptoms among 3,271 civilian survivors of the September 11, 2001, terrorist attacks on the World Trade Center. Am J Epidemiol 173(3):271–281.

Edelman P, Osterloh J, Pirkle J, Caudill SP, Grainger J, Jones R, Blount B, Calafat A, Turner W, Feldman D, Baron S, Bernard B, Lushniak BD, Kelly K, Prezant D [2003]. Biomonitoring of chemical exposure among New York City firefighters responding to the World Trade Center Fire and collapse. Environ Health Perspect 111(16):1906–1911.

Endara SM, Ryan MAK, Sevick CJ, Conlin AMS, Macera CA, Smith TC [2009]. Does acute maternal stress in pregnancy affect infant health outcomes? Examination of a large cohort of infants born after the terrorist attacks of September 11, 2001. BMC Public Health 9.

Engel SM, Berkowitz GS, Wolff MS, Yehuda R [2005]. Psychological trauma associated with the World Trade Center attacks and its effect on pregnancy outcome. Paediatr Perinat Epidemiol 19(5):334–341.

Farfel M, DiGrande L, Brackbill R, Prann A, Cone J, Friedman S, Walker DJ, Pezeshki G, Thomas P, Galea S, Williamson D, Frieden TR, Thorpe L [2008]. An overview of 9/11 experiences and respiratory and mental health conditions among World Trade Center Health Registry enrollees. J Urban Health 85(6):880–909.

Feldman DM, Baron SL, Bernard BP, Lushniak BD, Banauch G, Arcentales N, Kelly KJ, Prezant DJ [2004]. Symptoms, respirator use, and pulmonary function changes among New York City firefighters responding to the World Trade Center disaster. Chest 125(4):1256–1264.

Fireman EM, Lerman Y, Ganor E, Greif J, Fireman-Shoresh S, Lioy PJ, Banauch GI, Weiden M, Kelly KJ, Prezant DJ [2004]. Induced sputum assessment in New York City firefighters exposed to World Trade Center dust. Environ Health Perspect 112(15):1564–1569.

Galea S, Nandi A, Vlahov D [2005]. The epidemiology of post-traumatic stress disorder after disasters. Epidemiol Rev 27:78–91.

Galea S, Resnick H, Ahern J, Gold J, Bucuvalas M, Kilpatrick D, Stuber J, Vlahov D [2002]. Posttraumatic stress disorder in Manhattan, New York City, after the September 11th terrorist attacks. J Urban Health 79(3):340–353.

Galea S, Vlahov D, Resnick H, Ahern J, Susser E, Gold J, Bucuvalas M, Kilpatrick D [2003]. Trends of probable post-traumatic stress disorder in New York City after the September 11 terrorist attacks. Am J Epidemiol 158(6):514–524.

Gavett SH [2006]. Physical characteristics and health effects of aerosols from collapsed buildings. J Aerosol Med 19(1):84–91.

Gavett SH [2003]. World Trade Center fine particulate matter—chemistry and toxic respiratory effects: An overview. Environ Health Perspect 111(7):971.

Gavett SH, Haykal-Coates N, Highfill JW, Ledbetter AD, Chen LC, Cohen MD, Harkema JR, Wagner JG, Costa DL [2003]. World Trade Center fine particulate matter causes respiratory tract hyperresponsiveness in mice. Environ Health Perspect 111(7):981–991.

Geyh AS, Chillrud S, Williams DL, Herbstman J, Symons JM, Rees K, Ross J, Kim SR, Lim HJ, Turpin B, Breysse P [2005]. Assessing truck driver exposure at the World Trade Center disaster site: personal and area monitoring for particulate matter and volatile organic compounds during October 2001 and April 2002. J Occup Environ Hyg 2(3):179–193.

Grant X, Massa J, Ashwell L, Davis K, Schwab M, Geyh A [2007]. The World Trade Center Clean Up and Recovery Worker Cohort Study: Respiratory health amongst cleanup workers approximately 20 months after initial exposure at the disaster site. J Occup Environ Med 49(10):1063–1072.

Hall R, Trout D, Earnest G [2004]. An industrial hygiene survey of an office building in the vicinity of the World Trade Center: assessment of potential hazards following the collapse of the World Trade Center buildings. J Occup Environ Hyg *1*(5):D49–D53.

Henriksen CA, Bolton JM, Sareen J [2010]. The psychological impact of terrorist attacks: examining a dose-response relationship between exposure to 9/11 and Axis I mental disorders. Depress Anxiety *27*(11):993–1000.

Herbert R, Moline J, Skloot G, Metzger K, Baron S, Luft B, Markowitz S, Udasin I, Harrison D, Stein D, Todd A, Enright P, Stellman JM, Landrigan PJ, Levin SM [2006]. The World Trade Center disaster and the health of workers: five-year assessment of a unique medical screening program. Environ Health Perspect *114*(12):1853–1858.

Herbstman JB, Frank R, Schwab M, Williams DL, Samet JM, Breysse PN, Geyh AS [2005]. Respiratory effects of inhalation exposure among workers during the clean-up effort at the World Trade Center disaster site. Environ Res *99*(1):85–92.

Herbstman JB, Sjodin A, Kurzon M, Lederman SA, Jones RS, Rauh V, Needham LL, Tang D, Niedzwiecki M, Wang RY, Perera F [2010]. Prenatal exposure to PBDEs and neurodevelopment. Environ Health Perspect *118*(5):712–719.

Herdt-Losavio ML, Mauer MP, Carlson GA [2008]. Development of an exposure assessment method for epidemiological studies of New York State personnel who responded to the World Trade Center disaster. Ann Occup Hyg *52*(2):83–93.

Horii Y, Jiang Q, Hanari N, Lam PK, Yamashita N, Jansing R, Aldous KM, Mauer MP, Eadon GA, Kannan K [2010]. Polychlorinated dibenzo-p-dioxins, dibenzofurans, biphenyls, and naphthalenes in plasma of workers deployed at the World Trade Center after the collapse. Environ Sci Technol *44*(13):5188–5194.

Ilgren EB [2001]. Health risks from exposures to asbestos, metals, and various chemicals due to collapse of the World Trade Center: An environmental residential survey with a commentary related to Ground Zero workers. Indoor Built Environ *10*(6):361–383.

Izbicki G, Chavko R, Banauch GI, Weiden MD, Berger KI, Aldrich TK, Hall C, Kelly KJ, Prezant DJ [2007]. World Trade Center "sarcoid-like" granulomatous pulmonary disease in New York city fire department rescue workers. Chest *131*(5):1414–1423.

Johnson SB, Langlieb AM, Teret SP, Gross R, Schwab M, Massa J, Ashwell L, Geyh AS [2005]. Rethinking first response: Effects of the clean up and recovery effort on workers at the world trade center disaster site. J Occup Environ Med *47*(4):386–391.

Lall R, Ito K, Thurston GD [2011]. Distributed Lag Analyses of Daily Hospital Admissions and Source-Apportioned Fine Particle Air Pollution. Environ Health Perspect *119*(4):455–460.

Landrigan PJ, Forman J, Galvez M, Newman B, Engel SM, Chemtob C [2008]. Impact of September 11 World Trade Center disaster on children and pregnant women. Mt Sinai J Med 75(2):129–134.

Landrigan PJ, Lioy PJ, Thurston G, Berkowitz G, Chen LC, Chillrud SN, Gavett SH, Georgopoulos PG, Geyh AS, Levin S, Perera F, Rappaport SM, Small C, Grp NWTCW [2004]. Health and environmental consequences of the world trade center disaster. Environ Health Perspect 112(6):731–739.

Lange JH, Thomulka KW, Sites SLM, Priolo G, Mastrangelo G [2006]. Personal airborne asbestos exposure levels associated with various types of abatement. Bull Environ Contam Toxicol 76(3):389–391.

Laumbach RJ, Harris G, Kipen HM, Georgopoulos P, Shade P, Isukapalli SS, Efstathiou C, Galea S, Vlahov D, Wartenberg D [2009]. Lack of association between estimated World Trade Center plume intensity and respiratory symptoms among New York City residents outside of Lower Manhattan. Am J Epidemiol 170(5):640–649.

Lederman SA, Becker M, Sheets S, Stein J, Tang D, Weiss L, Perera FP [2008]. Modeling exposure to air pollution from the WTC disaster based on reports of perceived air pollution. Risk Anal 28(2):287–301.

Lederman SA, Jones RL, Caldwell KL, Rauh V, Sheets SE, Tang D, Viswanathan S, Becker M, Stein JL, Wang RY, Perera FP [2008]. Relation between cord blood mercury levels and early child development in a World Trade Center cohort. Environ Health Perspect 116(8):1085–1091.

Lederman SA, Rauh V, Weiss L, Stein JL, Hoepner LA, Becker M, Perera FP [2004]. The effects of the World Trade Center event on birth outcomes among term deliveries at three lower Manhattan hospitals. Environ Health Perspect 112(17):1772–1778.

Levin S, Herbert R, Skloot G, Szeinuk J, Teirstein A, Fischler D, Milek D, Piligian G, Wilk-Rivard E, Moline J [2002]. Health effects of World Trade Center site workers. Am J Ind Med 42(6):545–547.

Lin S, Gomez MI, Gensburg L, Liu W, Hwang SA [2010]. Respiratory and cardiovascular hospitalizations after the World Trade Center disaster. Arch Environ Occup Health 65(1):12–20.

Lin S, Jones R, Reibman J, Bowers J, Fitzgerald EF, Hwang SA [2007]. Reported respiratory symptoms and adverse home conditions after 9/11 among residents living near the World Trade Center. J Asthma 44(4):325–332.

Lin S, Jones R, Reibman J, Morse D, Hwang SA [2010]. Lower respiratory symptoms among residents living near the World Trade Center, two and four years after 9/11. Int J Occup Environ Health 16(1):44–52.

Lin S, Reibman J, Bowers JA, Hwang SA, Hoerning A, Gomez MI, Fitzgerald EF [2005]. Upper respiratory symptoms and other health effects among residents living near the world trade center site after September 11, 2001. Am J Epidemiol *162*(6):499–507.

Lioy PJ, Georgopoulos P [2006]. The anatomy of the exposures that occurred around the World Trade Center site: 9/11 and beyond. Ann N Y Acad Sci *1076*:54–79.

Lioy PJ, Pellizzari E, Prezant D [2006]. The World Trade Center aftermath and its effects on health: understanding and learning through human-exposure science. Environ Sci Technol *40*(22):6876–6885.

Lioy PJ, Weisel CP, Millette JR, Eisenreich S, Vallero D, Offenberg J, Buckley B, Turpin B, Zhong M, Cohen MD, Prophete C, Yang I, Stiles R, Chee G, et al. [2002]. Characterization of the Dust/Smoke Aerosol that Settled East of the World Trade Center (WTC) in Lower Manhattan after the Collapse of the WTC 11 September 2001. Environ Health Perspect *110*(7):703–714.

Lipkind HS, Curry AE, Huynh M, Thorpe LE, Matte T [2010]. Birth outcomes among offspring of women exposed to the september 11, 2001, terrorist attacks. Obstet Gynecol *116*(4):917–925.

Lippy BE [2002]. Safety and health of heavy equipment operators at Ground Zero. Am J Ind Med *42*(6):539–542.

Lorber M, Gibb H, Grant L, Pinto J, Pleil J, Cleverly D [2007]. Assessment of inhalation exposures and potential health risks to the general population that resulted from the collapse of the World Trade Center towers. Risk Anal *27*(5):1203–1221.

Lowers HA, Meeker GP, Lioy PJ, Lippmann M [2009]. Summary of the development of a signature for detection of residual dust from collapse of the World Trade Center buildings. J Expo Anal Environ Epidemiol *19*(3):325–335.

Malievskaya E, Rosenberg N, Markowitz S [2002]. Assessing the health of immigrant workers near Ground Zero: Preliminary results of the World Trade Center day laborer medical monitoring project. Am J Ind Med *42*(6):548–549.

Mann JM, Sha KK, Kline G, Breuer FU, Miller A [2005]. World Trade Center dyspnea: bronchiolitis obliterans with functional improvement: a case report. Am J Ind Med *48*(3):225–229.

Marmagas SW, King LR, Chuk MG [2003]. Public health's response to a changed world: September 11, biological terrorism, and the development of an environmental health tracking network. Am J Public Health *93*(8):1226–1230.

Mauer MP, Cummings KR [2010]. Impulse oscillometry and respiratory symptoms in World Trade Center responders, 6 years post-9/11. Lung *188*(2):107–113.

Mauer MP, Cummings KR, Carlson GA [2007]. Health effects in New York State personnel who responded to the World Trade Center disaster. J Occup Environ Med 49(11):1197–1205.

Mauer MP, Cummings KR, Hoen R [2010]. Long-term respiratory symptoms in World Trade Center responders. Occup Med (Lond) 60(2):145–151.

Mauer MP, Herdt-Losavio ML, Carlson GA [2010]. Asthma and lower respiratory symptoms in New York State employees who responded to the World Trade Center disaster. Int Arch Occup Environ Health 83(1):21–27.

McGee JK, Chen LC, Cohen MD, Chee GR, Prophete CM, Haykal-Coates N, Wasson SJ, Conner TL, Costa DL, Gavett SH [2003]. Chemical analysis of World Trade Center fine particulate matter for use in toxicologic assessment. Environ Health Perspect 111(7):972–980.

McMahon JT, Aslam R, Schell SE [2011]. Unusual ciliary abnormalities in three 9/11 response workers. Ann Otol Rhinol Laryngol 120(1):40–48.

Mendelson DS, Roggeveen M, Levin SM, Herbert R, de la Hoz RE [2007]. Air trapping detected on end-expiratory high-resolution computed tomography in symptomatic World Trade Center rescue and recovery workers. J Occup Environ Med 49(8):840–845.

Moline J, Herbert R, Nguyen N [2006]. Health consequences of the September 11 World Trade Center attacks: a review. Cancer Invest 24(3):294–301.

Moline JM, Herbert R, Crowley L, Troy K, Hodgman E, Shukla G, Udasin I, Luft B, Wallenstein S, Landrigan P, Savitz DA [2009]. Multiple Myeloma in World Trade Center Responders: A Case Series. J Occup Environ Med 51(8):896–902.

Moline JM, Herbert R, Levin S, Stein D, Luft BJ, Udasin IG, Landrigan PJ [2008]. WTC medical monitoring and treatment program: comprehensive health care response in aftermath of disaster. Mt Sinai J Med 75(2):67–75.

Nandi A, Galea S, Tracy M, Ahern J, Resnick H, Gershon R, Vlahov D [2004]. Job loss, unemployment, work stress, job satisfaction, and the persistence of posttraumatic stress disorder one year after the September 11 attacks. J Occup Environ Med 46(10):1057–1064.

Nawrot TS, Nemmar A, Nemery B [2007]. Update in environmental and occupational medicine 2006. Am J Respir Crit Care Med 175(8):758–762.

Ng SP, Dimitroulopoulou C, Grossinho A, Chen LC, Kendall M [2005]. PM2.5 exposure assessment of the population in Lower Manhattan area of New York City after the World Trade Center disaster. Atmos Environ 39(11):1979–1992.

Nolan RP, Ross M, Nord GL, Axten CW, Osleeb JP, Domnin SG, Price B, Wilson R [2005]. Risk assessment for asbestos-related cancer from the 9/11 attack on the World Trade Center. J Occup Environ Med 47(8):817–825.

Offenberg JH, Eisenreich SJ, Chen LC, Cohen MD, Chee G, Prophete C, Weisel C, Lioy PJ [2003]. Persistent organic pollutants in the dusts that settled across lower Manhattan after September 11, 2001. Environ Sci Technol 37(3):502–508.

Offenberg JH, Eisenreich SJ, Gigliotti CL, Chen LC, Xiong JQ, Quan CL, Lou XP, Zhong MH, Gorczynski J, Yiin LM, Illacqua V, Lioy PJ [2004]. Persistent organic pollutants in dusts that settled indoors in lower Manhattan after September 11, 2001. J Expo Anal Environ Epidemiol 14(2):164–172.

Ohlsson A, Shah PS [2011]. Effects of the September 11, 2001 disaster on pregnancy outcomes: A systematic review. Acta Obstet Gynecol Scand 90(1):6–18.

Olson DA, Norris GA [2008]. Chemical characterization of ambient particulate matter near the World Trade Center: Source apportionment using organic and inorganic source markers. Atmos Environ 42(31):7310–7315.

Olson DA, Norris GA, Landis M, Vette AF [2004]. Chemical characterization of ambient particulate matter near the world trade center: Elemental carbon, organic carbon, and mass reconstruction. Environ Sci Technol 38(17):4465–4473.

Olson DA, Norris GA, Seila RL, Landis MS, Vette AF [2007]. Chemical characterization of volatile organic compounds near the World Trade Center: Ambient concentrations and source apportionment. Atmos Environ 41(27):5673–5683.

Oppenheimer BW, Goldring RM, Herberg ME, Hofer IS, Reyfman PA, Liautaud S, Rom WN, Reibman J, Berger KI [2007]. Distal airway function in symptomatic subjects with normal spirometry following World Trade Center dust exposure. Chest 132(4):1275–1282.

Osinubi OYO, Gandhi SK, Ohman-Strickland P, Boglarsky C, Fiedler N, Kipen H, Robson M [2008]. Organizational factors and office workers' health after the World Trade Center terrorist attacks: Long-term physical symptoms, psychological distress, and work productivity. J Occup Environ Med 50(2):112–125.

Payne JP, Kemp SJ, Dewar A, Goldstraw P, Kendall M, Chen LC, Tetley TD [2004]. Effects of Airborne World Trade Center Dust on Cytokine Release by Primary Human Lung Cells In Vitro. J Occup Environ Med 46(5):420–427.

Perera F, Tang D, Whyatt R, Lederman SA, Jedrychowski W [2005]. DNA damage from polycyclic aromatic hydrocarbons measured by benzo[a]pyrene-DNA adducts in mothers and newborns from Northern Manhattan, the World Trade Center Area, Poland, and China. Cancer Epidemiol Biomarkers Prev 14(3):709–714.

Perera FP, Tang D, Rauh V, Lester K, Tsai WY, Tu YH, Weiss L, Hoepner L, King J, Del Priore G, Lederman SA [2005]. Relationships among polycyclic aromatic hydrocarbon-DNA adducts, proximity to the World Trade Center, and effects on fetal growth. Environ Health Perspect *113*(8):1062–1067.

Perera FP, Tang D, Rauh V, Tu YH, Tsai WY, Becker M, Stein JL, King J, Del Priore G, Lederman SA [2007]. Relationship between polycyclic aromatic hydrocarbon-DNA adducts, environmental tobacco smoke, and child development in the World Trade Center cohort. Environ Health Perspect *115*(10):1497–1502.

Perrin MA, DiGrande L, Wheeler K, Thorpe L, Farfel M, Brackbill R [2007]. Differences in PTSD Prevalence and Associated Risk Factors Among World Trade Center Disaster Rescue and Recovery Workers. Am J Psychiatry *164*(9):1385–1394.

Pleil JD, Funk WE, Rappaport SM [2006]. Residual indoor contamination from world trade center rubble fires as indicated by polycyclic aromatic hydrocarbon profiles. Environ Sci Technol *40*(4):1172–1177.

Pleil JD, Lorber MN [2007]. Relative congener scaling of Polychlorinated dibenzo-p-dioxins and dibenzofurans to estimate building fire contributions in air, surface wipes, and dust samples. Environ Sci Technol *41*(21):7286–7293.

Pleil JD, Vette AF, Johnson BA, Rappaport SM [2004]. Air levels of carcinogenic polycyclic aromatic hydrocarbons after the World Trade Center disaster. Proc Natl Acad Sci U S A *101*(32):11685–11688.

Prezant DJ, Weiden M, Banauch GI, McGuinness G, Rom WN, Aldrich TK, Kelly KJ [2002]. Cough and bronchial responsiveness in firefighters at the world trade center site. N Engl J Med *347*(11):806–815.

Pulcino T, Galea S, Ahern J, Resnick H, Foley M, Vlahov D [2003]. Posttraumatic stress in women after the September 11 terrorist attacks in New York City. J Womens Health *12*(8):809–820.

Qureshi S, Dutkiewicz VA, Khan AR, Swami K, Yang KX, Husain L, Schwab JJ, Demerjian KL [2006]. Elemental composition of PM2.5 aerosols in Queens, New York: Solubility and temporal trends. Atmos Environ *40*:S238–S251.

Rayne S [2005]. Using exterior building surface films to assess human exposure and health risks from PCDD/Fs in New York City, USA, after the World Trade Center attacks. J Hazard Mater *127*(1–3):33–39.

Rayne S, Ikonomou MG, Butt CM, Diamond ML, Truong J [2005]. Polychlorinated dioxins and furans from the World Trade Center attacks in exterior window films from lower Manhattan in New York City. Environ Sci Technol *39*(7):1995–2003.

Reibman J, Lin S, Hwang SA, Gulati M, Bowers JA, Rogers L, Berger KI, Hoerning A, Gomez M, Fitzgerald EF [2005]. The World Trade Center residents' respiratory health study: new-onset respiratory symptoms and pulmonary function. Environ Health Perspect *113*(4):406–411.

Reibman J, Liu M, Cheng Q, Liautaud S, Rogers L, Lau S, Berger KI, Goldring RM, Marmor M, Fernandez-Beros ME, Tonorezos ES, Caplan-Shaw CE, Gonzalez J, Filner J, Walter D, Kyng K, Rom WN [2009]. Characteristics of a residential and working community with diverse exposure to World Trade Center dust, gas, and fumes. J Occup Environ Med *51*(5):534–541.

Rom WN, Reibman J, Rogers L, Weiden MD, Oppenheimer B, Berger K, Goldring R, Harrison D, Prezant D [2010]. Emerging exposures and respiratory health: World Trade Center dust. Proc Am Thorac Soc *7*(2):142–145.

Rom WN, Weiden M, Garcia R, Ting AY, Vathesatogkit P, Tse DB, McGuinness G, Roggli V, Prezant D [2002]. Acute eosinophilic pneumonia in a New York City firefighter exposed to World Trade Center dust. Am J Respir Crit Care Med *166*(6):797–800.

Safirstein BH, Klukowicz A, Miller R, Teirstein A [2003]. Granulomatous pneumonitis following exposure to the World Trade Center collapse. Chest *123*(1)301–304.

Salzman SH, Moosavy FM, Miskoff JA, Friedmann P, Fried G, Rosen MJ [2004]. Early respiratory abnormalities in emergency services police officers at the World Trade Center site. J Occup Environ Med *46*(2):113–122.

Samet JM, Geyh AS, Utell MJ [2007]. The legacy of World Trade Center dust. N Engl J Med *356*(22):2233–2236.

Skloot G, Goldman M, Fischler D, Goldman C, Schechter C, Levin S, Teirstein A [2004]. Respiratory symptoms and physiologic assessment of ironworkers at the World Trade Center disaster site. Chest *125*(4):1248–1255.

Skloot GS, Schechter CB, Herbert R, Moline JM, Levin SM, Crowley LE, Luft BJ, Udasin IG, Enright PL [2009]. Longitudinal assessment of spirometry in the World Trade Center medical monitoring program. Chest *135*(2):492–498.

Stellman JM, Smith RP, Katz CL, Sharma V, Charney DS, Herbert R, Moline J, Luft BJ, Markowitz S, Udasin I, Harrison D, Baron S, Landrigan PJ, Levin SM, Southwick S [2008]. Enduring mental health morbidity and social function impairment in world trade center rescue, recovery, and cleanup workers: the psychological dimension of an environmental health disaster. Environ Health Perspect *116*(9):1248–1253.

Swartz E, Stockburger L, Vallero DA [2003]. Polycyclic aromatic hydrocarbons and other semivolatile organic compounds collected in New York City in response to the events of 9/11. Environ Sci Technol *37*(16):3537–3546.

Szeinuk J, Padilla M, de la Hoz RE [2008]. Potential for diffuse parenchymal lung disease after exposures at World Trade Center Disaster site. Mt Sinai J Med 75(2):101–107.

Szema AM, Khedkar M, Maloney PF, Takach PA, Nickels MS, Patel H, Modugno F, Tso AY, Lin DH [2004]. Clinical deterioration in pediatric asthmatic patients after September 11, 2001. J Allergy Clin Immunol 113(3):420–426.

Szema AM, Savary KW, Ying BL, Lai K [2009]. Post 9/11: High asthma rates among children in Chinatown, New York. Allergy Asthma Proc 30(6):605–611.

Tang KM, Nace CG, Jr., Lynes CL, Maddaloni MA, LaPosta D, Callahan KC [2004]. Characterization of background concentrations in upper Manhattan, New York apartments for select contaminants identified in World Trade Center dust. Environ Sci Technol 38(24):6482–6490.

Tao L, Kannan K, Aldous KM, Mauer MP, Eadon GA [2008]. Biomonitoring of perfluorochemicals in plasma of New York State personnel responding to the World Trade Center disaster. Environ Sci Technol 42(9):3472–3478.

Tao X, Massa J, Ashwell L, Davis K, Schwab M, Geyh A [2007]. The World Trade Center Clean Up and Recovery Worker Cohort Study: Respiratory Health Amongst Cleanup Workers Approximately 20 Months After Initial Exposure at the Disaster Site. J Occup Environ Med 49(10):1063–1072.

Tapp LC, Baron S, Bernard B, Driscoll R, Mueller C, Wallingford K [2005]. Physical and mental health symptoms among NYC transit workers seven and one-half months after the WTC attacks. Am J Ind Med 47(6):475–483.

Thayer WC, Griffith DA, Diamond GL [2007]. Geography of asbestos contamination near the World Trade Center site. Stoch Env Res Risk A 21(5):461–471.

Thomas PA, Brackbill R, Thalji L, DiGrande L, Campolucci S, Thorpe L, Henning K [2008]. Respiratory and other health effects reported in children exposed to the World Trade Center disaster of 11 September 2001. Environ Health Perspect 116(10):1383–1390.

Trout D, Nimgade A, Mueller C, Hall R, Earnest GS [2002]. Health effects and occupational exposures among office workers near the World Trade Center disaster site. J Occup Environ Med 44(7):601–605.

Udasin I, Schechter C, Crowley L, Sotolongo A, Gochfeld M, Luft B, Moline J, Harrison D, Enright P [2011]. Respiratory symptoms were associated with lower spirometry results during the first examination of WTC responders. J Occup Environ Med 53(1):49–54.

Wagner VL, Radigan MS, Roohan PJ, Anarella JP, Gesten FC [2005]. Asthma in Medicaid managed care enrollees residing in New York City: results from a post-World Trade Center disaster survey. J Urban Health 82(1):76–89.

Wallingford KM, Snyder EM [2001]. Occupational exposures during the World Trade Center disaster response. Toxicol Ind Health 17(5–10):247–253.

Wanahita N, See JL, Giedd KN, Friedmann P, Somekh NN, Bergmann SR [2010]. No Evidence of Increased Prevalence of Premature Coronary Artery Disease in New York City Police Officers as Predicted by Coronary Artery Calcium Scoring. J Occup Environ Med 52(6):661–665.

Wang S, Prophete C, Soukup JM, Chen LC, Costa M, Ghio A, Qu QS, Cohen MD, Chen HB [2010]. Roles of MAPK pathway activation during cytokine induction in BEAS-2B cells exposed to fine World Trade Center (WTC) dust. J Immunotoxicol 7(4):298–307.

Webber MP, Gustave J, Lee R, Niles JK, Kelly K, Cohen HW, Prezant DJ [2009]. Trends in respiratory symptoms of firefighters exposed to the world trade center disaster: 2001–2005. Environ Health Perspect 117(6):975–980.

Weiden MD, Ferrier N, Nolan A, Rom WN, Comfort A, Gustave J, Zeig-Owens R, Zheng S, Goldring RM, Berger KI, Cosenza K, Lee R, Webber MP, Kelly KJ, Aldrich TK, Prezant DJ [2010]. Obstructive airways disease with air trapping among firefighters exposed to World Trade Center dust. Chest 137(3):566–574.

Wolff MS, Teitelbaum SL, Lioy PJ, Santella RM, Wang RY, Jones RL, Caldwell KL, Sjodin A, Turner WE, Li W, Georgopoulos P, Berkowitz GS [2005]. Exposures among pregnant women near the World Trade Center site on 11 September 2001. Environ Health Perspect 113(6):739–748.

Wu M, Gordon RE, Herbert R, Padilla M, Moline J, Mendelson D, Litle V, Travis WD, Gil J [2010]. Case report: Lung disease in World Trade Center responders exposed to dust and smoke: carbon nanotubes found in the lungs of World Trade Center patients and dust samples. Environ Health Perspect 118(4):499–504.

Xu A, Prophete C, Chen LC, Emala CW, Cohen MD [2011]. Interactive Effect of Cigarette Smoke Extract and World Trade Center Dust Particles on Airway Cell Cytotoxicity. J Toxicol Environ Health A 74(14):887–902.

Yehuda R, Cai G, Golier JA, Sarapas C, Galea S, Ising M, Rein T, Schmeidler J, Muller-Myhsok B, Holsboer F, Buxbaum JD [2009]. Gene Expression Patterns Associated with Posttraumatic Stress Disorder Following Exposure to the World Trade Center Attacks. Biol Psychiatry 66(7):708–711.

Yiin LM, Millette JR, Vette A, Ilacqua V, Quan CL, Gorczynski J, Kendall M, Chen LC, Weisel CP, Buckley B, Yang I, Lioy PJ [2004]. Comparisons of the dust/smoke particulate that settled inside the surrounding buildings and outside on the streets of southern New York city after the collapse of the World Trade Center, September 11, 2001. J Air Waste Manage Assoc 54(5):515–528.

B. Editorials, Abstracts, News Articles (Not Peer-Reviewed)

Dangerous dust: WTC residue & long-term health problems. [2002]. Emerg Med Serv 31(11):56.

Physical health status of World Trade Center rescue and recovery workers and volunteers—New York City, July 2002–August 2004. [2004]. MMWR Morb Mortal Wkly Rep 53(35):807–812.

Potential Exposures to Airborne and Settled Surface Dust in Residential Areas of Lower Manhattan Following the Collapse of the World Trade Center—New York City, November 4–December 11, 2001. [2003]. MMWR Morb Mortal Wkly Rep 52(7):131–136.

Ahern J, Galea S, Resnick H, Vlahov D [2004]. The longitudinal course of probable PTSD following the September 11 terrorist attacks. Am J Epidemiol 159(11):S89–S89.

Aldous K [2003]. Chemical analysis related to the World Trade Center terrorist attack. Abstr Pap Am Chem Soc 226:003–SOCED.

ATSDR, Health NYCDo [2003]. Final Technical Report of the Public Health Investigation to Assess Potential Exposures to Airborne and Settled Surface Dust in Residential Areas of Lower Manhattan. [http://www.atsdr.cdc.gov/asbestos/asbestos/types_of_exposure/_downloads/final-report-lowermanhattan-02-execsummary.pdf]. Date accessed 06/25/2011.

Ault A [2004]. World Trade Center rescuers face lung distress. Lancet 363(9421):1614.

Banauch G, Weiden N, Hall C, Cohen HW, Aldrich TK, Arcentales N, Kelly KJ, Prezant DJ [2005]. Accelerated pulmonary function decline after World Trade Center particulate exposure in the New York City Fire Department workforce. Chest 128(4):213S–213S.

Banauch GI, Dhala A, Prezant DJ [2005]. Pulmonary disease in rescue workers at the World Trade Center site. Curr Opin Pulm Med 11(2):160–168.

Beckett WS [2002]. A New York City firefighter—Overwhelmed by World Trade Center dust. Am J Respir Crit Care Med 166(6):785–786.

Berkowitz G, Wolff M, Janevic T, Holzman I, Landrigan P [2003]. The World Trade Center disaster and intrauterine growth restriction. Am J Epidemiol 157(11):266.

Bernard B, Driscoll R, Baron S, Wallingford K, Mueller C [2007]. Health hazard evaluation report: HETA-2002–0090; 2002–0096; 2002–0101–3028, Buildings in the Vicinity of the World Trade Center, New York City, New York. [http://www.cdc.gov/niosh/hhe/reports/pdfs/2002-0101-3028.pdf]. Date accessed 06/25/2011.

Bernard BP, Baron SL, Mueller CA, Driscoll RJ, Tapp LC, Wallingford KM, Tepper AL [2002]. Impact of September 11 attacks on workers in the vicinity of the World Trade Center—New York City. MMWR Morb Mortal Wkly Rep 52(SP):8–10.

Betts K [2010]. Signature of high exposure to WTC toxics identified. Environ Sci Technol 44(13):4834–4835.

Betts K [2002]. WTC dust may cause respiratory problems. World Trade Center. Environ Sci Technol 36(13):273A.

Borkowski JB [2003]. Chemical, biological and radiation detection in the immediate aftermath of the WTC collapse. Abstr Pap Am Chem Soc 226:180-ANYL.

Brackbill R, DiGrande L, team W [2006]. Adverse health impacts and injuries in survivors of collapsed and damaged buildings on 9/11 - World Trade Center Health Registry (WTCHR). Am J Epidemiol 163(11):S242–S242.

Brackbill RM, Thorpe LE, DiGrande L, Perrin M, Sapp JH, 2nd, Wu D, Campolucci S, Walker DJ, Cone J, Pulliam P, Thalji L, Farfel MR, Thomas P [2006]. Surveillance for World Trade Center disaster health effects among survivors of collapsed and damaged buildings. MMWR Surveill Summ 55(2):1–18.

Breysse PN, Williams DA, Henshaw S, Rees K, Herbstman J, Symons JM, Watson M, Geyh A [2002]. Asbestos exposures to truck drivers during World Trade Center clean up operations. Epidemiology 13(4):238.

Burton A [2010]. Lung damage lingers after 9/11. Environ Health Perspect 118(6):A245.

Cahill TA, Cliff SS, Perry KD, Bench GS, Leifer R [2003]. Very fine particles from the WTC collapse piles: Anaerobic incineration? Abstr Pap Am Chem Soc 226:108–ENVR.

Cahill TA, Cliff SS, Shackelford JF, Kelly PB, Bench G, Perry KD [2002]. Aerosols from the World Trade Center collapse site. Abstr Pap Am Chem Soc 224:161–PHYS.

Chen L, Cohen M, Maciejczyk P, Cohen B, Heikkinen M, Kendall M, Lippmann M, Costa M, Thurston G [2002]. Characterization of the World Trade Center disaster airborne and settled particulate matter. Epidemiology 13(4):243.

Chillrud SN, Geyh A, Ross J, Wallace S, Ramstrom S, Spengler JD, Breysse P, Kinney PL [2002]. Comparing World Trade Center (WTC) related exposures of particulate bound metals to levels measured in the NYC teach study. Epidemiology 13(4):240.

Chillrud SN, Geyh AS, Levy DK, Chettiar EM, Chaky DA [2003]. World Trade Center Environmental Contaminant Database: A publicly available air quality dataset for the New York City area. Abstr Pap Am Chem Soc 226:137-ENVR.

Clark RN [2002]. USGS Environmental Studies of the World Trade Center Area, New York City, after September 11, 2001. Date accessed 06/25/2011.

Clark RN, Green RO [2001]. Environmental studies of the World Trade Center area after the September 11, 2001 attack. Date accessed 06/25/2011.

Claudio L [2003]. Firefighter findings. Environ Health Perspect 111(16):A896.

Cohen BS, Heikkinen MSA, Hazi Y [2003]. Fine and ultrafine partices near the World Trade Center disaster site. Abstr Pap Am Chem Soc 226:114-ENVR.

Crouch EA, Green LC [2007]. Comment on "Persistent organic pollutants in 9/11 world trade center rescue workers: reduction following detoxification" by James Dahlgren, Marie Cecchini, Harpreet Takhar, and Olaf Paepke [Chemosphere 69/8 (2007) 1320-1325]. Chemosphere 69(8):1330-1332; discussion 1333-1336.

Dahlgren J, Cecchini M, Takhar H, Paepke O [2007]. Reply to comment of Edmund A.C. Crouch and Laura C. Green, on: "Persistent organic pollutants in 9/11 World Trade Center rescue workers: Reduction following detoxification" by James Dahlgren, Marie Cecchini, Harpreet Takhar, and Olaf Paepke Chemosphere 69/8 (2007) 1320-1325. Chemosphere 69(8):1333-1336.

de la Hoz RE [2010]. Long-term outcomes of acute irritant-induced asthma and World Trade Center-related lower airway disease. Am J Respir Crit Care Med 181(1):95-96.

de la Hoz RE [2010]. Occupational asthma and lower airway disease among World Trade Center workers and volunteers. Curr Allergy Asthma Rep 10(4):287-294.

de la Hoz RE [2011]. Occupational lower airway disease in relation to World Trade Center inhalation exposure. Curr Opin Allergy Clin Immunol 11(2):97-102.

de la Hoz RE, Shohet MR, Cohen JM [2010]. Occupational rhinosinusitis and upper airway disease: the world trade center experience. Curr Allergy Asthma Rep 10(2):77-83.

Dorea JG [2009]. Cord blood mercury and early child development: effects of the World Trade Center. Environ Health Perspect 117(1):A14; author reply A14-15.

Elder A, Finkelstein J, Gelein R, Corson N, Mercer P, Reed C, Oakes D, Eberly S, Topham D, Oberdorster G [2004]. In vitro and in vivo effects of world trade center dusts: studies in human and mouse cell lines and in influenza-compromised young and old rats. Toxicologist 78(1-S):288.

EPA [2003]. Interim Final WTC Residential Confirmation Cleaning Study [http://www.epa.gov/wtc/reports/confirmation_cleaning_study.pdf]. Date accessed 06/25/2011.

EPA [2003]. Summary Report of the U.S. EPA Technical Peer Review Meeting on the Draft Document Entitled: Exposure and Human Health Evaluation of Airborne Pollution from the World Trade Center Disaster. EPA/600/R-03/142

EPA [2002]. Toxicological Effects of Fine Particulate Matter Derived from the Destruction of the World Trade Center. [http://www.epa.gov/nheerl/wtc/WTC_report_7b3i.pdf]. Date accessed 06/25/2011.

EPA [2003]. World Trade Center Background Study Report Interim Final. [http://www.epa.gov/wtc/reports/background_study_report.pdf]. Date accessed 06/25/2011.

EPA [2003]. World Trade Center Indoor Environment Assessment: Selecting Contaminants of Potential Concern and Setting Health-Based Benchmarks. [http://www.epa.gov/wtc/reports/contaminants_of_concern_benchmark_study.pdf]. Date accessed 06/25/2011.

EPA [2005]. World Trade Center Residential Dust Cleanup Program. [http://www.epa.gov/wtc/reports/residential_dust_cleanup_final_report.pdf]. Date accessed 06/25/2011.

Feldman DM, Edelman P, Baron S, Mueller C, Bernard B, Lushniak BD, Kelly KJ, Prezant DJ [2002]. Health effects, respirator use and biomonitoring results among New York City firefighters responding to the World Trade Center (WTC) disaster - September, 2001. Am J Epidemiol *155*(11):L6.

Ferrier N, Nolan A, Rom WN, Comfort AL, Prezant DJ, Weiden MD [2010]. Similar exposure to World Trade Center (WTC) dust produced variable lung function decline: defining most and least effected subgroups in the FDNY cohort. Am J Respir Crit Care Med *181*(1):A1252.

Gavett SH, Haykal-Coates N, Chen L, Cohen MD, Costa DL [2003]. Respiratory toxicological effects of world trade center fine particulate matter in mice. Toxicol Sci *72*:287.

Georgopoulos PG [2003]. Plume reconstruction and microenvironmental modeling for assessing exposures to contaminants associated with the WTC fire and collapse. Toxicol Sci *72*:285.

Geyh A, Tao XG, Gross R, Massa J, Ashwell L, Zybert P, Herman D, Langlieb A, Breysse P [2004]. Health effects among workers involved in the clean up and recovery effort at the World Trade Center (WTC) disaster site: The WTC clean up and recovery workers health. Epidemiology *15*(4):S123–S124.

Geyh AS, Chillrud S, Williams D, Herbstman J, Symons J, Watson M, Breysse P [2003]. Exposure assessment of workers involved in cleanup operations at the World trade Center disaster site. Toxicol Sci 72:286.

Geyh AS, Chillrud S, Williams DA, Herbstman J, Symons JM, Watson M, Breysse P [2002]. Exposure assessment of workers in the clean up operation at the World Trade Center Disaster Site. Epidemiology 13(4):239.

Gibbs L, Farley T, Aldrich TK, Chen LC, Gelberg KH, Kleinman EJ, Klitzman S, Landrigan PJ, Leinhardt RR, Prezant D, Raju R, Reibman J, Slone MS, Thorpe L [2009]. 2009 annual report on 9/11 health. 2009 Annual Report on 9/11 Health:1–24.

Gibbs L, Farley T, Aldrich TK, Cohen M, Difede J, Gelberg KH, Greene C, Kleinman EJ, Landrigan PJ, Leinhardt RR, Prezant D, Raju R, Reibman J, Sadler P, Slone MS [2010]. 2010 annual report on 9/11 health. 2010 Annual Report on 9/11 Health:1–14.

Gibbs L, Frieden TR, Aldrich TK, Chen LC, Gelberg KH, Kleinman EJ, Klitzman S, Landrigan PJ, Leinhardt RR, Marshall RD, Prezant D, Raju R, Reibman J, Rosin D, Slone MS, Thorpe L [2008]. 2008 annual report on 9/11 health. 2008 Annual Report on 9/11 Health:1–25.

Grant LD, Pinto JP, Galizia A [2003]. Approaches to evaluation of potential human exposures and health impacts associated with airborne contaminants from world trade center collapse/fires. Toxicol Sci 72:288.

Hall RM, Trout D, Earnest GS, Mueller C, Nimgade A [2002]. Health hazard evaluation report: HETA-2002-0038-2870, 26 Federal Plaza, New York, New York. [http://www.cdc.gov/niosh/hhe/reports/pdfs/2002-0038-2870.pdf]. Date accessed 06/25/2011.

Hanson BL, Sztern B, Lange JH, Prezant D, Weiden M, Kelly KJ [2003]. Cough and bronchial responsiveness in firefighters at the world trade center site. N Engl J Med 348 (1):76–77.

Harley NH, Chittaporn P, Kong A, Fisenne IM [2005]. Airborne Pb-210 particle size measurements during and after the WTC collapse. Health Phys 89(1):S30–S30.

Harville E, Xiong X, Buekens P [2010]. Disasters and perinatal health: A systematic review. Obstet Gynecol Surv 65(11):713–728.

Hazi Y, Chillrud SN, Maciejczyk P [2003]. Mass and elemental composition of size segregated airborne particulate matter near the World Trade Center disaster site. Abstr Pap Am Chem Soc 226:131–ENVR.

Heikkinen MSA, Hsu SI, Lall R, Peters PA, Cohen BS, Chen LC, Thurston G [2003]. Aerosol measurements at the WTC site one year after. Abstr Pap Am Chem Soc 226:132–ENVR.

Herbert R, Skloot G, Metzger K, Landrigan PJ, Moline J, Stein D, Todd A, Levin SM, Baron S, Udasin I [2007]. WTC five-year assessment: Herbert et al. respond. Environ Health Perspect 115(2):A72–A73.

Herbstman J, Frank R, Schwab M, Samet J, Breysse P, Geyh A [2002]. Predicting pulmonary function in rubble removal workers at the World Trade Center Disaster Site. Epidemiology 13(4):237.

Herbstman J, Schwab M, Samet J, Breysse P, Geyh A [2002]. Respiratory health symptoms in rubble removal workers at the World Trade Center disaster site: Descriptive results. Epidemiology 13(4):236.

Howard J [2008]. The 9/11 World Trade Center disaster: past and future. Mt Sinai J Med 75(2):65–66.

Huynh M, Maslow C, Pezeshki G, Friedman S [2008]. Dust cloud exposure during the world trade center attack and lower respiratory symptoms in lower Manhattan residents. Am J Epidemiol 167(11):S105–S105.

Kahn HD, Santella D [2010]. Comment on: "Summary of the development of a signature for the detection of residual dust from collapse of the World Trade Center buildings". J Expo Sci Environ Epidemiol 20(4):393–394.

Kapalka G, Letizia G, Bascom R, Qian ZM, Buyantseva L, Young M, Roberts A [2004]. Physical and mental health of New York City police officers 18 months after the World Trade Center attacks. Epidemiology 15(4):S123–S123.

Kendall M, Breger D, Chen LC [2002]. SEM characterization of WTC plume particles: Indoor airborne and deposited dust. Epidemiology 13(4):241.

Kligler B [2006]. Why publish the Olive Leaf Report? Explore (NY) 2(5):399.

Kokayi K, Altman CH, Callely RW, Harrison A [2006]. Findings of and treatment for high levels of mercury and lead toxicity in ground zero rescue and recovery workers and lower Manhattan residents. Explore (NY) 2(5):400–407.

Lange JH [2003]. Cough and bronchial responsiveness in firefighters at the World Trade Center site. N Engl J Med 348(1):76–77; author reply 76–77.

Lange JH [2001]. Has the World Trade Center tragedy established a new standard for asbestos? Indoor Built Environ 10(6):346–349.

Lange JH [2003]. Health effects of local residents near the World Trade Center: Have they been forgotten? J Occup Environ Med 45(5):465–466.

Lange JH [2002]. How do you interpret regulations: through science or agency rules? Toxicol Ind Health 18(2):107–108.

Leifer R, Bench G, Cahill T [2003]. Characterization of plumes passing over lower Manhattan after the WTC disaster. Abstr Pap Am Chem Soc 226:254-ENVR.

Leon WJ, Bowler R, Haseeb MA, Hansard PC [2003]. Clinical and psychological abnormalities in New York City police officers who served at the World Trade Center (WTC) disaster site. Chest 124(4):215S-215S.

Levin SM, Herbert R, Moline J [2006]. Health effects among World Trade Center responders. Lung Cancer 54:36.

Lin S [2008]. Methodology Challenges and Strategies on Assessing Respiratory Health Among the Residents Living Near the Former World Trade Center. Epidemiology 19(6):S48-S48.

Lin S, Reibman J, Bowers J, Hwang SA, Gomez M, Fitzgerald E [2004]. Upper respiratory symptoms and other health effects among the residents living near the former world trade center after the September 11 disaster. Epidemiology 15(4):S127-S127.

Lin S, Reibman J, Jones RR, Hwang SA, Hoerning A, Gomez MI, Fitzgerald EF [2005]. Lin et al. respond to "Assessment of respiratory symptoms after September 11". Am J Epidemiol 162(6):511-512.

Lioy PJ, Collaborators NE [2003]. Overview of the conditions lending to exposures that resulted from the collapse and fires at The World Trade Center. Abstr Pap Am Chem Soc 226:106-ENVR.

Lioy PJ, Gochfeld M [2002]. Lessons learned on environmental, occupational, and residential exposures from the attack on the World Trade Center. Am J Ind Med 42(6):560-565.

Lowers HA, Meeker GP, Brownfield IK [2005]. Analysis of Background Residential Dust for World Trade Center Signature Components Using Scanning Electron Microscopy and X-ray Microanalysis. [http://pubs.usgs.gov/of/2005/1073/]. Date accessed 06/25/2011.

Lubick N [2008]. WTC responders have high blood levels of perfluorinated compounds. Environ Sci Technol 42(9):3123.

Maa M, Kazeros A, Turetz ML, Parsia SS, Caplan Shaw CE, Walter D, Liu M, Rogers L, Marmor M, Reibman J [2010]. Peripheral eosinophils are associated with new onset and persistent wheezing and dyspnea in World Trade Center exposed individuals. Am J Respir Crit Care Med 181(1):A4691.

Maciejczyk P, Zeisler R, Hwang JS, Thurston GD, Chen LC [2003]. Characterization of size-fractionated World Trade Center dust and estimation of relative dust contribution to ambient concentrations. Abstr Pap Am Chem Soc 226:109-ENVR.

Maddaloni MA [2003]. Indoor air assessment for the world trade center site: Selecting contaminants of potential concern and setting health-based benchmarks. Toxicol Sci 72:289.

Malo JL, Gautrin D, Martin J [2003]. Irritant-induced asthma: epidemiology and pathogenesis. NIOSH Final Grant Report. PB2005-105203

Manetti Cusa J, Cohen I, Varma S, Caplan Shaw CE, Kazeros A, Parsia SS, Turetz M, Liu M, Walter D, Marmor M, Reibman J [2010]. Persistent respiratory symptoms are a risk factor for mental health symptoms in residents and workers exposed to world trade center dust, gas and fumes presenting for medical care. Am J Respir Crit Care Med 181(1):A4688.

Manuel JS [2001]. NIEHS responds to World Trade Center attacks. Environ Health Perspect 109(11):A526–527.

McKinney K, Benson S, Lempert A, Singal M, Wallingford K, Snyder E [2002]. Occupational exposures to air contaminants at the World Trade Center disaster site—New York, September–October, 2001. MMWR Morb Mortal Wkly Rep 51(21):453–456.

Meeker G, Plumlee G, Sutley S, Lamothe P, Ziegler T, Swayze G, Hoefen T, Clark R, Brownfield I, Gent C, Lowers H [2003]. Microanalysis and chemical characterization of ousts generated by the World Trade Center collapse. Abstr Pap Am Chem Soc 226:133-ENVR.

Meeker GP, Bern AM, Lowers HA, Brownfield IK [2005]. Determination of a Diagnostic Signature for World Trade Center Dust Using Scanning Electron Microscopy Point Counting Techniques. [http://pubs.usgs.gov/of/2005/1031/]. Date accessed 06/25/2011.

Meeker GP, Lioy PJ, Lippmann M, Lowers HA [2010]. Response to the comment by Henry Kahn and Dennis Santella on a summary of the development of a signature for detection of residual dust from the collapse of the World Trade Center buildings. J Expo Anal Environ Epidemiol 20(6):491–492.

Miller A [2009]. Asthma following the 2001 World Trade Center attack. JAMA 302(21):2319; author reply 2319–2320.

Miller A [2008]. Incidence of new onset asthma after the World Trade Center disaster. Environ Health Perspect 116(7):A286.

Miller A [2007]. Limitations of WTC five-year assessment. Environ Health Perspect 115(2):A71–72; author reply A72–73.

Miller A [2007]. Sarcoidosis, firefighters sarcoidosis, and world trade center "Sarcoid-Like" granulomatous pulmonary disease. Chest 132(6):2053–2053.

Miller A [2009]. World Trade Center Multiple Myeloma: Police Responders Only? J Occup Environ Med 51(12):1357–1357.

Miller A, Mann J [2009]. Longitudinal assessment of spirometry in World Trade Center responders. Chest 136(4):1182–1183; author reply 1183.

Moline JM, Herbert R, Crowley L, Troy K, Hodgman E, Shukla G, Udasin I, Luft B, Wallenstein S, Landrigan P, Savitz DA [2009]. World Trade Center Multiple Myeloma: Police Responders Only? Response. J Occup Environ Med 51(12):1357–1358.

Nemery B [2003]. Reactive fallout of World Trade Center dust. Am J Respir Crit Care Med 168(1):2–3.

Nemery B [2004]. World Trade Center dust and airway reactivity. Am J Respir Crit Care Med 169(7):885–885.

NIOSH [2002]. Protecting workers at the World Trade Center site. Response from the National Institute for Occupational Safety and Health. [http://www.cdc.gov/niosh/02-143.html]. Date accessed 06/25/2011.

Parekh P, Semkow T, Husain L, Haines D, Wozniak G [2006]. Tritium in the World Trade Center September 11th, 2001 Terrorist Attack: It's Possible Sources and Fate. [https://e-reports-ext.llnl.gov/pdf/240430.pdf]. Date accessed 06/25/2011.

Parekh P, Semkow TM, Husain L, Wozniak GJ [2002]. Tritium in the World Trade Center Disaster: Its possible sources and fate. Abstr Pap Am Chem Soc 223:026–NUCL.

Perera F, Rauh V, Wyatt R, Lederman S, Miller R, Jedrychowski W, Kinney P, Camann D, Andrews H, Orjuela M, Tang D [2007]. International research on the effects of in utero exposure to air pollutants on child growth and development, asthma, and cancer risk. Epidemiology 17(6)(Suppl):S412.

Perrin MA [2008]. Ms. Perrin replies. Am J Psychiatry 165(2):262.

Pinto JP, Grant LD, Huber AH, Vette AF [2003]. Evaluation of potential human exposures and health impacts of airborne particulate matter (PM) and its constituents following the collapse of the World Trade Center towers. Abstr Pap Am Chem Soc 226:136–ENVR.

Platner J [2002]. Industrial hygiene at the World Trade Center disaster. Appl Occup Environ Hyg 17(2):84–85.

Plumlee GS, Hageman PL, Meeker GP, Lamothe PJ, Theodorakos P, Sutley SJ, Clark RN, Wilson SA, Swayze GA, Hoefen TM, Taggart J, Adams M, Ziegler TL [2003]. The chemical composition and reactivity of dusts deposited by the 9/11/2001, World Trade Center collapse. Toxicol Sci 72:925.

Prezant D, Kelly K, Jackson B, Peterson D, Feldman D, Baron S, Mueller CA, Bernard B, Lushniak B, Smith L, BerryAnn R, Hoffman B [2002]. Use of respiratory protection among responders at the World Trade Center site—New York City, September 2001. MMWR Morb Mortal Wkly Rep 51(SP):6–8.

Prezant DJ, Banauch GI [2004]. World Trade Center dust and airway reactivity. Am J Respir Crit Care Med 169(7):884–884.

Qian ZM, Robert G, Buyantseva L, Enright P, Kapalka G, Young M, Roberts A, Pogash R [2004]. Acute respiratory responses to September 11: A survey of 446 New York police officers. Epidemiology 15(4):S121–S122.

Scanlon PD [2002]. World Trade Center cough—A lingering legacy and a cautionary tale. N Engl J Med 347(11):840–842.

Selco JI, Riddle SG, Kelly PB, Cahill TA [2002]. Mass spectrometric analysis of aerosol particulates from the World Trade Center. Abstr Pap Am Chem Soc 224:194–PHYS.

Semkow TM, Hafner RS, Parekh PP, Wozniak GJ, Haines DK, Husain L, Rabun RL, Williams PG [2002]. Elevated tritium levels at the World Trade Center. [http://www.escholarship.org/uc/item/4xq88667]. Date accessed 06/25/2011.

Service RF [2003]. World Trade Center. Chemical studies of 9/11 disaster tell complex tale of 'bad stuff'. Science 301(5640):1649.

Skloot [2009]. Longitudinal Assessment of Spirometry in the World Trade Center Medical Monitoring Program (vol 135, pg 492, 2009). Chest 135(4)(Correction):1114–1114.

Skloot GS, Enright PL [2009]. Longitudinal Assessment of Spirometry in World Trade Center Responders Response. Chest 136(4):1183–1183.

Smith RP, Katz CL, Holmes A, Herbert R, Levin S, Moline J, Landsbergis P, Stevenson L, North CS, Larkin GL, Baron S, Hurrell Jr JJ [2004]. Mental health status of World Trade Center rescue and recovery workers and volunteers - New York City, July 2002 - August 2004. MMWR Morb Mortal Wkly Rep 53(35):812–815.

Stephenson J [2002]. Researchers probe health consequences following the World Trade Center attack. JAMA 288(10):1219–1221.

Swartz E, Stockburger L, Vallero D [2002]. Monitoring toxic organic gases and particles near the world trade center after September 11, 2001. Epidemiology 13(4):233.

Szema AM, Khedkar M, Maloney PF, Takach PA, Nickels MS, Patel H, Modugno F, Tso AY, Lin DH, Chen HT [2004]. Clinic record review of pediatric asthmatic patients after September 11, 2001, does not support authors' conclusions - Reply. J Allergy Clin Immunol 114(4):989–990.

Tao X, Massa J, Ashwell L, Davis K, Schwab M, Geyh A [2006]. The world trade center clean up and recovery worker cohort study: Respiratory health among clean up workers approximately 20 months after initial exposure at the disaster site. Epidemiology 17(6):S512–S513.

Tapp L, Wallingford K, Mueller C, Baron S [2005]. Health hazard evaluation report: HETA-2002-0095-2955, Metropolitan Transit Authority of New York City, New York City, New York. [http://www.cdc.gov/niosh/hhe/reports/pdfs/2002-0095-2955.pdf]. Date accessed 06/25/2011.

Thomas PA, Brackbill R, Thalji L, Campolucci S, DiGrande L, Thorpe L, Stellman SD, Henning K [2009]. World Trade Center Disaster and Asthma Type: Thomas et al. Respond. Environ Health Perspect 117(2):A57–A57.

Thurston G, Maciejczyk P, Lall R, Hwang JS, Chen LC [2003]. Identification and characterization of World Trade Center disaster fine particulate matter air pollution at a site in lower manhattan following September 11. Epidemiology 14(5):S87–S88.

Thurston GD, Maciejczyk P, Lall R, Hwang JS, Hsu SI, Chen LC [2003]. Nature and impact of World Trade Center disaster fine particulate matter air pollution at a site in Lower Manhattan after September 11. Abstr Pap Am Chem Soc 226:134–ENVR.

Trout DB [2003]. Health effects of local residents near the World Trade Center: Have they been forgotten? Reply. J Occup Environ Med 45(5):466–466.

Truncale T, Brooks S, Prezant DJ, Banauch GI, Nemery B [2004]. World Trade Center dust and airway reactivity. Am J Respir Crit Care Med 169(7):883–884; author reply 884–885.

Vette A, Landis M, Swartz E, Williams R, LaPosta D, Kantz M, Filippelli J, Webb L, Ellestad T, Vallero D [2002]. Concentration and speciation of PM at ground zero and lower Manhattan following the collapse of the WTC. Epidemiology 13(4):235.

Vlahov D, Galea S [2005]. Invited commentary: Considering bias in the assessment of respiratory symptoms among residents of Lower Manhattan following the events of September 11, 2001. Am J Epidemiol 162(6):508–510.

Washam C [2008]. Asthma among WTC children: registry yields first child health report. Environ Health Perspect 116(10):A440.

Weiden MD, Ferrier N, Nolan A, Rom WN, Comfort A, Gustave J, Zheng S, Goldring R, Berger K, Cosenza K, Beringer A, Glass L, Lee R, Zeig Owens R, Webber M, Prezant DJ [2009]. World Trade Center collapse produced airway injury and air trapping. Am J Respir Crit Care Med 179(1):A5852.

Weisel CP, Lioy PJ, Millette J, Eisenreich S, Vallero D, Offenberg J, Buckley B, Turpin B, Zhong M, Cohen MD, Prophete C, Yang I, Stiles R, Chee G, Johnson W, Alimokhtari S, Weschler C, Chen LC [2002]. Characterization of the dust/smoke aerosol that settled east of the World Trade Center (WTC) after it's collapse. Epidemiology *13*(4):234.

Wolff MS, Teitelbaum SL, Lioy PJ, Santella RM, Georgopoulos P, Li W, Berkowitz GS [2004]. Exposures among pregnant women near the World Trade Center site on 9/11. Epidemiology *15*(4)S120–S120.

Ziem G [2009]. World Trade Center disaster and asthma type. Environ Health Perspect *117*(2):A56–57.

Appendix C. Cancer-Related Publications and Articles

A. Peer-Reviewed Publications

Moline J, Herbert R, Nguyen N [2006]. Health consequences of the September 11 World Trade Center attacks: a review. Cancer Invest 24(3):294–301.

Moline JM, Herbert R, Crowley L, Troy K, Hodgman E, Shukla G, Udasin I, Luft B, Wallenstein S, Landrigan P, Savitz DA [2009]. Multiple myeloma in World Trade Center responders: a case series. J Occup Environ Med 51(8):896–902.

Nolan RP, Ross M, Nord GL, Axten CW, Osleeb JP, Domnin SG, Price B, Wilson R [2005]. Risk assessment for asbestos-related cancer from the 9/11 attack on the World Trade Center. J Occup Environ Med 47(8):817–825.

Rayne S [2005]. Using exterior building surface films to assess human exposure and health risks from PCDD/Fs in New York City, USA, after the World Trade Center attacks. J Hazard Mater 127(1–3):33–39.

Samet JM, Geyh AS, Utell MJ [2007]. The legacy of World Trade Center dust. N Engl J Med 356(22):2233–2236.

B. Editorial Letters

Miller A [2009]. World Trade Center multiple myeloma: police responders only? J Occup Environ Med 51(12):1357; author reply 1357–1358.

Moline JM, Herbert R, Crowley L, Troy K, Hodgman E, Shukla G, Udasin I, Luft B, Wallenstein S, Landrigan P, Savitz DA [2009]. World Trade Center multiple myeloma: police responders only? Response. J Occup Environ Med 51(12):1357–1358.

C. Abstracts, Articles Mentioning Cancer, and Student Thesis

de la Hoz RE, Shohet MR, Cohen JM [2010]. Occupational rhinosinusitis and upper airway disease: the world trade center experience. Curr Allergy Asthma Rep 10(2):77–83.

Hitt E [2001]. The World Trade Center attack and cancer risk: a waiting game. Lancet Oncology 2(11):652–652.

Perera F, Rauh V, Whyatt R, Lederman S, Miller R, Jedrychowski W, Kinney P, Camann D, Andrews H, Orjuela M, Tang D [2006]. International research on the effects of in utero exposure to air pollutants on child growth and development, asthma, and cancer risk. Epidemiology 17(6):S412–S412.

Soares BD [2010]. Analysis of potential mutagenic effects of World Trade Center dust on in vitro systems.

Appendix D. Cancer Classification Systems

A. IARC Monographs on the Evaluation of Carcinogenic Risks to Humans[13]

The International Agency for Research on Cancer (IARC) is part of the World Health Organization and follows the general governing rules of the UN family of organizations, but is governed by its own governing bodies. IARC's mission is to coordinate and conduct research on the causes of human cancer and the mechanisms of carcinogenesis, and to develop scientific strategies for cancer prevention and control. The Agency is involved in both epidemiological and laboratory research and disseminates scientific information through publications, meetings, courses, and fellowships. One of IARC's scientific products is a series of Monographs which critically review and evaluate the available evidence on the carcinogenicity of a wide range of human exposures. Through the Monographs program, IARC seeks to identify the causes of human cancer.

Agents are selected for review on the basis of two main criteria: (a) there is evidence of human exposure and (b) there is some evidence or suspicion of carcinogenicity. Each Monograph reviews exposure data and other information on an agent under consideration as well as all pertinent epidemiological studies and cancer bioassays in experimental animals. Mechanistic and other relevant data are also reviewed. In the Monographs, an agent is termed 'carcinogenic' if it is capable of increasing the incidence of malignant neoplasms, reducing their latency, or increasing their severity or multiplicity. The induction of benign neoplasms may contribute to the judgment that the agent is carcinogenic. In addition to studies that support a finding of a cancer hazard, the Monograph evaluations also consider studies that do not.

Several groups may attend Monograph development meetings. The Working Group is responsible for the critical reviews and evaluations that are developed during the meeting. Invited Specialists are experts who also have critical knowledge and experience but have a real or apparent conflict of interests. Representatives of national and international health agencies often attend meetings, but do not participate in the evaluations. Observers with relevant scientific credentials may be admitted to a meeting by IARC in limited numbers. The IARC Secretariat consists of scientists who are designated by IARC and who have relevant expertise. They serve as rapporteurs and participate in all discussions.

Approximately one year in advance of the meeting of a Working Group, the agents to be reviewed are announced on the Monographs program website (http://monographs.iarc.fr) and participants are selected by IARC staff in consultation with other experts.

---

[13]Description based on http://monographs.iarc.fr/ENG/Preamble/CurrentPreamble.pdf.

Relevant biological and epidemiological data are collected by IARC from recognized sources of information on carcinogenesis, including data storage and retrieval systems such as PubMed. Meeting participants who are asked to prepare preliminary working papers for specific sections are expected to supplement the IARC literature searches with their own searches. The Working Group meets at IARC to discuss and finalize the texts and to formulate the evaluations. IARC Working Groups strive to achieve a broad consensus evaluation, but not necessarily unanimity.

Several types of epidemiological study contribute to the assessment of carcinogenicity in humans: cohort studies, case–control studies, correlation (or ecological) studies, and intervention studies. Rarely, results from randomized trials may be available. Case reports and case series of cancer in humans may also be reviewed.

The evidence relevant to carcinogenicity from studies in humans is classified into one of the following categories: (1) Sufficient evidence of carcinogenicity; (2) Limited evidence of carcinogenicity; (3) Inadequate evidence of carcinogenicity; or (4) Evidence suggesting lack of carcinogenicity.

The evidence relevant to carcinogenicity in experimental animals is classified into one of the following categories: (1) Sufficient evidence of carcinogenicity; (2) Limited evidence of carcinogenicity; (3) Inadequate evidence of carcinogenicity; (4) Evidence suggesting lack of carcinogenicity.

Mechanistic and other evidence judged to be relevant to an evaluation of carcinogenicity and of sufficient importance to affect the overall evaluation is highlighted in the Monographs. This may include data on pre-neoplastic lesions, tumor pathology, genetic and related effects, structure–activity relationships, metabolism and toxicokinetics, physicochemical parameters, and analogous biological agents.

Finally, the body of evidence is considered as a whole, in order to reach an overall evaluation of the carcinogenicity of the agent to humans. The agent is described according to the wording of one of the following categories, and the designated group is given. The categorization of an agent is a matter of scientific judgment that reflects the strength of the evidence derived from studies in humans and in experimental animals and from mechanistic and other relevant data.

Group 1. Carcinogenic to Humans

This category is used when there is sufficient evidence of carcinogenicity in humans. Exceptionally, an agent may be placed in this category when evidence of carcinogenicity in humans is less than sufficient, but there is sufficient evidence of carcinogenicity in experimental animals and strong evidence in exposed humans that the agent acts through a relevant mechanism of carcinogenicity.

Group 2A. Probably Carcinogenic to Humans

This category is used when there is limited evidence of carcinogenicity in humans and sufficient evidence of carcinogenicity in experimental animals. In some cases, an agent may be classified in this category when there is inadequate evidence of carcinogenicity in humans and sufficient evidence of carcinogenicity in experimental animals and strong evidence that the carcinogenesis is mediated by a mechanism that also operates in humans. Exceptionally, an agent may be classified in this category solely on the basis of limited evidence of carcinogenicity in humans. An agent may be assigned to this category if it clearly belongs, based on mechanistic considerations, to a class of agents for which one of more members have been classified in Group A or in Group 2A.

Group 2B. Possibly Carcinogenic in Humans

This category is used for agents for which there is limited evidence of carcinogenicity in humans and less than sufficient evidence of carcinogenicity in experimental animals. It may also be used when there is inadequate evidence of carcinogenicity in experimental animals. In some instances, an agent for which there is inadequate evidence for carcinogenicity in humans and less than sufficient evidence of carcinogenicity in experimental animals together with supporting evidence from mechanistic and other relevant data may be placed in this group. An agent may be classified in this category solely on the basis of strong evidence from mechanistic and other relevant data.

Group 3. Not Classifiable as to Its Carcinogenicity to Humans

This category is used most commonly for agents for which the evidence of carcinogenicity is inadequate in humans and inadequate or limited in experimental animals. Exceptionally, agents for which the evidence of carcinogenicity is inadequate in humans but sufficient in experimental animals may be placed in this category when there is strong evidence that the mechanism of carcinogenicity in experimental animals does not operate in humans. Agents that do not fall into any other group are also placed in this category. An evaluation in Group 3 is not a determination of non-carcinogenicity or overall safety. It often means that further research is needed, especially when exposures are widespread or the cancer data are consistent with differing interpretations.

Group 4. Probably Not Carcinogenic to Humans

This category is used for agents for which there is evidence suggesting lack of carcinogenicity in humans and in experimental animals. In some instances, agents for which there is inadequate evidence of carcinogenicity in humans, but evidence suggesting lack of carcinogenicity in experimental animals, consistently and strongly supported by a broad range of mechanistic and other relevant data, may be classified in this group.

B. U.S. National Toxicology Program Report on Carcinogens[14]

The National Toxicology Program (NTP) Report on Carcinogens (RoC) is an informational scientific and public health document that identifies and discusses agents, substances, mixtures, or exposure circumstances that may pose a hazard to human health by virtue of their carcinogenicity. The RoC is published biennially and serves as a meaningful and useful compilation of data on:

1. Carcinogenicity, genotoxicity, and biologic mechanisms of the listed substance in humans and/or animals;
2. Potential for human exposure to these substances; and
3. Federal regulations to limit exposures.

The RoC is mandated by Section 301(b)(4) of the Public Health Services Act, as amended, which stipulates that the Secretary of the Department of Health and Human Services shall publish the report which contains:

1. A list of all substances (i) which either are known to be carcinogens [in humans] or may reasonably be anticipated to be [human] carcinogens; and (ii) to which a significant number of persons residing in the United States are exposed;
2. Information concerning the nature of such exposure and the estimated number of persons exposed to such substances;
3. A statement identifying (i) each substance contained in this list for which no effluent, ambient, or exposure standard has been established by a Federal agency; and (ii) for each effluent, ambient, or exposure standard established by a Federal agency with respect to a substance contained in this list, the extent to which, on the basis of available medical, scientific, or other data, such standard, and the implementation of such standard by the agency, decreases the risk to public health from exposure to the substance; and
4. A description of (i) each request received during the year to conduct research into, or testing for, the carcinogenicity of substances and (ii) how the Secretary and each such other entity, respectively, have responded to each request.

Nominations for listing or removing in the RoC are obtained from various sources, including: periodic requests from the public through Federal Register notices, the NTP Update newsletter, and other appropriate publications; active solicitations from member agencies of the NTP Executive Committee; from reviews of the literature performed by the NTP; identification from sources such as the NTP Technical Reports, the IARC Monographs on the Evaluation of the Carcinogenic Risk of Chemicals to Humans, the California Environmental Protection Agency's Carcinogen List, and other similar

---

[14] The description is based on the NTP website found at: http://ntp.niehs.nih.gov/?objectid=72016262-BDB7-CEBA-FA60E922B18C2540 and is relevant to the NTP 12th Report on Carcinogens.

sources. The RoC is required to list only substances to which a significant number of people living in the United States are exposed; therefore, substances to which very few people are exposed are generally not listed.

Much of the information on specific chemicals or occupational exposures has been published in the scientific literature or in publicly available and peer-reviewed technical reports. The scientific literature and publicly available and peer-reviewed technical reports are a primary source of information for identifying and evaluating substances for listing in the RoC. Many of the listed substances also have been reviewed and evaluated by other organizations, including the IARC in Lyon, France, the Environmental Protection Agency of the State of California, and other U.S. Federal and international agencies.

Both human and laboratory animal studies are used to evaluate whether substances are possible human carcinogens. The strongest evidence for establishing a relationship between exposure to any given substance and cancer in humans comes from epidemiological studies. The long-term animal bioassay is another valuable method for identifying substances as potential human carcinogens.

The nominations for listing in, or delisting from, the RoC are evaluated by two Federal scientific review groups and one non-governmental scientific peer-review body (a standing subcommittee of the NTP Board of Scientific Counselors). Each group reviews the relevant data on the carcinogenicity of the substances nominated and the exposure of U.S. residents to the substances. Public comment is solicited after the determination is made by the Director of the National Institute of Environmental Health Sciences (NIEHS) to review a nomination, after the two Federal scientific review groups have made their recommendations to the Director, and again after the non-governmental scientific peer-review body has reviewed the nominations and made a recommendation to the Director.

The NTP Director received the independent recommendations of the two Federal scientific review groups and one non-governmental scientific peer-review body, the opinion of the NTP Executive Committee, and all public comments concerning the nominations. The NTP Director evaluated this input and any other relevant information on the nominations and developed recommendations to the Secretary, DHHS, regarding whether to list or not to list the nominations in the RoC. Upon approval of the RoC, the Secretary submitted it to the U. S. Congress as a final document.

Two important new elements in the 12th RoC review process are (1) the public peer review of draft background documents by ad hoc scientific expert panels and (2) the public peer review of draft substance profiles by the NTP Board of Scientific Counselors. In addition, the NTP will, on a trial basis, prepare a response to public comments for the 12th RoC.

The RoC does not present quantitative assessments of the risks of cancer associated with these substances. Thus listing of substances in the RoC only indicates a potential hazard and does not establish the exposure conditions that would pose cancer risks to individuals in their daily lives. The substances listed in the RoC are either known or reasonably anticipated to cause cancer in humans in certain situations. With many listed substances, cancer may develop only after prolonged exposure. The criteria for listing an agent, substance, mixture, or exposure circumstance in the RoC are as follows:

- **Known to be a human carcinogen**

  There is sufficient evidence of carcinogenicity from studies in humans and indicates a causal relationship between exposure to the agent, substance, or mixture, and human cancer.

- **Reasonably anticipated to be a human carcinogen**

  There is limited evidence of carcinogenicity from studies in humans, and indicates that causal interpretation is credible, but that alternative explanations, such as chance, bias, or confounding factors, could not adequately be excluded; or

  There is sufficient evidence of carcinogenicity from studies in experimental animals, which indicates there is an increased incidence of malignant and/or a combination of malignant and benign tumors (1) in multiple species or at multiple tissue sites, or (2) by multiple routes of exposure, or (3) to an unusual degree with regard to incidence, site, or type of tumor, or age at onset; or

  There is less than sufficient evidence of carcinogenicity in humans or laboratory animals; however, the agent, substance, or mixture belongs to a well-defined, structurally related class of substances whose members are listed in a previous RoC as either known to be a human carcinogen or reasonably anticipated to be a human carcinogen, or there is convincing relevant information that the agent acts through mechanisms indicating it would likely cause cancer in humans.

Conclusions regarding carcinogenicity in humans or experimental animals are based on scientific judgment, with consideration given to all relevant information. Relevant information includes, but is not limited to, dose response, route of exposure, chemical structure, metabolism, pharmacokinetics, sensitive sub-populations, genetic effects, or other data relating to mechanism of action or factors that may be unique to a given substance. For example, there may be substances for which there is evidence of carcinogenicity in laboratory animals, but there are compelling data indicating that the agent acts through mechanisms which do not operate in humans and would therefore not reasonably be anticipated to cause cancer in humans.

Appendix E. IARC and NTP Designations for Identified Chemical Agents

Table 3. IARC and NTP designations for identified chemical agents

Agent	IARC[15]	NTP[16]
(E)-2-(6-Nonexnoxy)-tetrahydropyran	NL	NL
1,1,1-Trichloroethane	3	NL
1,1,2,2-Tetrachloroethane	3	NL
1,1,2-Trichloroethane	3	NL
1,1-Dichloroethane	NL	NL
1,1-Dichloroethylene	3	NL
1,2,3-Triphenyl-3-vinyl-cyclopropene	NL	NL
1,2,4-Trichlorobenzene	NL	NL
1,2,4-Trimethylbenzene	NL	NL
1,2-Dibromoethane	2A	B
1,2-Dichlorobenzene	3	NL
1,2-Dichloroethane	2B	B
1,2-Dichloropropane	3	NL
1,3,5-Trimethylbenzene	NL	NL
1,3-Butadiene	1	A
1,3-Dichlorobenzene	3	NL
1,3-Dichloropropane	NL	NL
1,4-Dichlorobenzene	2B	B
1,4-Dioxane	2B	B
12-Acetoxydaphnetoxin	NL	NL
1-Azabicyclo[2.2.2]octan-3-one	NL	NL
1-Dodecanol,2-methyl-,(S)-	NL	NL
1H-1,2,4-Triazole,1-ethyl	NL	NL
1-Heptene	NL	NL
1-Hexadecanol,2-methyl	NL	NL

See footnotes at end of table.

(Continued)

IARC and NTP designations for identified chemical agents (Continued)

Agent	IARC[15]	NTP[16]
1-Hexyl-2-nitrocyclohexane	NL	NL
1H-Indene,1-(phenylmethylene)-	NL	NL
1H-Pyrrole-3-propanoic acid,2,5-dihydro-4-methyl-2,5-dioxo	NL	NL
1-Hydroxypyrene	NL	NL
1-Methylanthracene	NL	NL
1-Methylnaphthalene	NL	NL
1-Methylphenanthrene	3	NL
1-Pentacontanol	NL	NL
2-(3'-Hydroxyphenylamino)-5-methyl-4-oxo-3,4-dihydropyrimidine	NL	NL
2,3,4-Trimethylhexane	NL	NL
2,3-Dihydrofluoranthene	NL	NL
2,3-Dimethyl-1-pentanol	NL	NL
2,4,5-Trichlorophenol	2B	NL
2,4,6-Trichlorophenol	2B	B
2,4-Dichlorodiphenyltrichloroethane	2B	NL
2,4-Dichlorophenol	2B	NL
2,4-Dimethylheptane	NL	NL
2,4-Dimethylhexane	NL	NL
2,4-Dimethylphenol	NL	NL
2,4-Dinitrophenol	NL	NL
2,4-Dinitrotoluene	2B	NL
2,4-Toluenediisocyanate	2B	B
2,6-Dimethylnaphthalene	NL	NL
2,6-Dinitrotoluene	2B	NL
2,6-Toluenediisocyanate	2B	NL
2-Benzylquinoline	NL	NL
2-Butanone	NL	NL

See footnotes at end of table.

(Continued)

IARC and NTP designations for identified chemical aents (Continued)

Agent	IARC[15]	NTP[16]
2-Chloronaphthalene	NL	NL
2-Chlorophenol	2B	NL
2-Hexanone	NL	NL
2-Hexyl-1-decanol	NL	NL
2-Methylnaphthalene	NL	NL
2-Methylphenol	NL	NL
2-Nitroaniline	NL	NL
2-Nitrophenol	NL	NL
3,3'-Dichlorobenzidine	2B	B
3,3-Dimethylhexane	NL	NL
3,4-Dihydrocyclopenta(cd)pyrene	3	NL
3-Chloropropylene	3	NL
3-Methoxycarbonyl-2-methyl-5-(2,3,5-tri-O-acetyl-beta-d-ribofuranosyl)	NL	NL
3-Nitroaniline	NL	NL
4,4'-Biphenyldicarbonitrile	NL	NL
4,6-Dinitro-2-methylphenol	NL	NL
4-Bromophenylether	NL	NL
4-Chloro-3-methylphenol	NL	NL
4-Chloroaniline	2B	NL
4-Chlorophenyl-phenylether	NL	NL
4-Ethyltoluene	NL	NL
4-Hydroxymandelic acid	NL	NL
4-Methyl-2-propyl-1-pentanol	NL	NL
4-Methylphenanthrene	NL	NL
4-Methylphenol	NL	NL
4-Nitroaniline	NL	NL
4-Nitrophenol	NL	NL

See footnotes at end of table.

(Continued)

IARC and NTP designations for identified chemical agents (Continued)

Agent	IARC[15]	NTP[16]
7-Methyl-3,4,5(2H)-tetrahydroazepine	NL	NL
9,10-Anthraquinone	NL	NL
9H-Fluorene,9-(phenylmethylene)	NL	NL
Acenaphthene	3	NL
Acenaphthylene	NL	NL
Acetone	NL	NL
Acrylonitrile	2B	B
Aldrin	3	NL
Aluminum	NL	NL
Anthracene	3	NL
Antimony	NL	NL
Antimony trioxide	2B	NL
Antimony trisulfide	3	NL
Arsenic	1	A
Asbestos	1	A
Auraptenol	NL	NL
Barium	NL	NL
Benzaldehyde	NL	NL
N-acetyl-Benzamide	NL	NL
Benzene Hexachloride	2B	B
Benzene	1	A
1,1'-(1,3-butadiyne-1,4-diyl)bis-benzene	NL	NL
Benzimidazo[2,1-a]isoquinoline	NL	NL
Benzo(a)anthracene	2B	B
Benzo(a)pyrene	1	B
Benzo(b)fluoranthene	2B	B
Benzo(e)pyrene	3	NL
Benzo(g,h,l)perylene	3	NL

See footnotes at end of table.

(Continued)

IARC and NTP designations for identified chemical agents (Continued)

Agent	IARC[15]	NTP[16]
Benzo(k)fluoranthene	2B	2
Benzyl alchohol	NL	NL
Benzyl butyl phthalate	3	NL
Benzyl chloride	2A	NL
Beryllium	1	A
Biphenyl	NL	NL
bis(2-Chloroethoxy)methane	NL	NL
bis(2-Chloroethyl)ether	3	NL
bis(2-Chloroisopropyl)ether	NL	NL
bis(2-Ethylhexyl)phthalate	3	B
Bismuth	NL	NL
Brominated diphenyl ethers	NL	NL
Bromobenzene	NL	NL
Bromodichloromethane	2B	B
Bromoform	3	NL
Bromomethane	3	NL
Cadmium	1	A
Calcite	NL	NL
Calcium	NL	NL
Carbazole	3	NL
Carbon disulfide	NL	NL
Carbon tetrachloride	2B	B
Cellulose	NL	NL
Cesium	NL	NL
Chlordane	2B	NL
Chloride(s)	NL	NL
Chlorobenzene	NL	NL
Chlorodifluoromethane	3	NL
Chloroethane	3	NL

See footnotes at end of table.

(Continued)

IARC and NTP designations for identified chemical agents (Continued)

Agent	IARC[15]	NTP[16]
Chloroform	2B	B
Chloromethane	3	NL
Chromium	Metal 3, III 3, VI 1	VI A
Chrysene	2B	NL
Chrysotile asbestos	1	A
cis-1,2-dichloroethylene	NL	NL
cis-1,3-dichloropropylene	NL	NL
Cobalt (see cobalt metal with tungsten carbide 2A, cobalt metal without tungsten carbide 2B, and cobalt sulfate and other soluble cobalt(II) salts 2B	varies with type	SULFATE B
Copper	NL	NL
Cycloate	NL	NL
Cyclohexane	NL	NL
Cyclohexanemethanol	NL	NL
Decachlorobiphenyl	NL	NL
Dibenzo(a)anthracene	2B	B
Dibenzo(a,h)anthracene	2A	B
Dibenzofuran	NL	NL
Dibenzothiophene	NL	NL
Dibromochloromethane	3	NL
Dibromomethane	NL	NL
Dibutyl phthalate	NL	NL
Dichlorodifluoromethane	NL	NL
Dichlorotetrafluoroethane	NL	NL
Dicyclohexylphthalate	NL	NL
Didodecylphthalate	NL	NL
Dieldrin	3	NL
Diethylphthalate	NL	NL
Dihydrogeraniol	NL	NL

See footnotes at end of table.

(Continued)

IARC and NTP designations for identified chemical agents (Continued)

Agent	IARC[15]	NTP[16]
Diisobutylphthalate	NL	NL
Dimethylcyanamide	NL	NL
Dimethylphthalate	NL	NL
Di-n-octylphthalate	NL	NL
Droserone(2,8-dihydroxy-3-methyl-1,4-naphthoquinone)	NL	NL
Endosulfan (I)	NL	NL
Endosulfan (II)	NL	NL
Endosulfan sulfate	NL	NL
Endrin	NL	NL
Endrin aldehyde	NL	NL
Endrin ketone	NL	NL
Ethanol	NL	NL
Ethyl acetate	NL	NL
Ethylbenzene	2B	NL
Fluoranthene	3	NL
Fluorene	3	NL
Fluoride	NL	NL
Formaldehyde	1	A
Gallium	NL	NL
Gypsum	NL	NL
Halite	NL	NL
Heptachlor	2B	NL
Heptachlor epoxide	NL	NL
Hexachlorobenzene	2B	B
Hexachlorobutadiene	3	NL
Hexachlorocyclopentadiene	NL	NL
Hexachloroethane	2B	B
Hexamethylene diisocyanate	NL	NL

See footnotes at end of table.

(Continued)

IARC and NTP designations for identified chemical agents (Continued)

Agent	IARC[15]	NTP[16]
Hexyl_N-butyrate	NL	NL
Hexylpentyl ether	NL	NL
Hydrogen bromide	NL	NL
Hydrogen chloride	3	NL
Hydrogen cyanide	NL	NL
Hydrogen fluoride	NL	NL
Indeno(1,2,3-cd)pyrene	2B	B
1-Propylbenzene	NL	NL
Iron	1	NL
Isopentane	NL	NL
Isophorone	NL	NL
Isophorone diisocyanate	NL	NL
Isopropyl alcohol	3	NL
Isopropylbenzene	NL	NL
Lead	Inorganic 2A Organic 3	B
Lithium	NL	NL
Magnesium	NL	NL
Manganese	NL	NL
Mercury	METALLIC AND INORGANIC Hg 3	NL
Methoxychlor	NL	NL
Methyl isobutyl ketone	NL	NL
Methyl tert-butyl ether	NL	NL
Methylalpha-ketopalmitate	NL	NL
Methylcyclopentane	NL	NL
Methylene chloride	2B	B
Methylstyrene	3	NL
Metribuzin	NL	NL

See footnotes at end of table. (Continued)

IARC and NTP designations for identified chemical agents (Continued)

Agent	IARC[15]	NTP[16]
Mica	NL	NL
Mirex	2B	B
Molybdenum	NL	NL
Monobutylphthalate	NL	NL
Naphthalene	2B	B
Naphthalene, 1-(methylthio)-	NL	NL
Naphthalene, 1,3-dimethylene	NL	NL
n-Butane	NL	NL
Nefopam	NL	NL
n-Heptane	NL	NL
n-Hexane	NL	NL
Nickel	METAL 2B CMPDS 1	METAL B CMPDS A
Nitrate	INGESTED 2A	NL
Nitric acid	NL	NL
Nitric oxide	NL	NL
Nitrobenzene	2B	B
Nitrogen dioxide	NL	NL
N-Nitroso-Di-n-propylamine	2B	B
N-Nitrosodiphenylamine	3	NL
n-Octane	NL	NL
n-Pentane	NL	NL
Ozone	NL	NL
p,p'-Dichlorodiphenyldichloroethane	2B	NL
p,p'-Dichlorodiphenyldichloroethylene	2B	NL
p,p'-Dichlorodiphenyltrichloroethane	2B	B
Pentachlorophenol	2B	NL
Pentanoicacid,4,4-dimethyl-3-methylene-,ethylester	NL	NL
Phenanthrene	3	NL

See footnotes at end of table.

(Continued)

IARC and NTP designations for identified chemical agents (Continued)

Agent	IARC[15]	NTP[16]
Phenol	3	NL
Phosphoric acid	NL	NL
Phthalate	NL	NL
Phthalic_acid, 2-hexylester	NL	NL
Polychlorinated biphenyls	2A	B
Portlandite	NL	NL
Potassium	NL	NL
Prometryn (caparol)	NL	NL
Propane	NL	NL
Propylene	3	NL
Pyrene	3	NL
Quartz	1	A
Quartz (Cristobalite)	1	A
Quartz (Tridymite)	1	A
Rubidium	NL	NL
Selenium	3	SULFIDE B
Silver	NL	NL
Sodium	NL	NL
Stress	2B	NL
Strontium	Sr-90 1	NL
Styrene	2B	B
Sulfate	NL	NL
Sulfur dioxide	3	NL
Sulfuric Acid	1	A
Synthetic vitreous fibers	Glass filament 3	B
Tetrachloroethylene	2A	B
Tetrahydrofuran	NL	NL
Thallium	NL	NL
Titanium	DIOXIDE 2B	NL

See footnotes at end of table.

(Continued)

IARC and NTP designations for identified chemical agents (Continued)

Agent	IARC[15]	NTP[16]
Toluene	3	NL
Toxaphene	2B	B
trans-1,2-Dichloroethylene	NL	NL
trans-1,3-Dichloropropylene	NL	NL
Trichloroethylene	2A	B
Trichlorofluoromethane	NL	NL
Trichlorotrifluoroethane	NL	NL
Uranium	NL	NL
Vanadium	PENTOXIDE 1	NL
Vernolate(vernam)	NL	NL
Vinyl acetate	2B	NL
Vinyl chloride	1	A
Xanthene	NL	NL
Xylene (o-,m-,p-)	3	NL
Zinc	NL	NL

[15]IARC categories are described in Appendix D, part A.
[16]NTP Categories are: A: Known to be a human carcinogen and B: Reasonably anticipated to be a human carcinogen. Descriptions of these categories are provided in Appendix D, part B.

www.ingramcontent.com/pod-product-compliance
Lightning Source LLC
Chambersburg PA
CBHW080307180526
45167CB00006B/2701